PUBLIC HEALTH IN THE 21ST CENTURY

MORE PRESCRIPTION FOR CHANGE

CASE STUDIES FOR APPLICATIONS OF STRATEGY AND STRATEGIC INTERVENTION IN NATIONAL AND INTERNATIONAL HEALTH SYSTEMS IN RESPONSE TO A COVID PANDEMIC

PUBLIC HEALTH IN THE 21ST CENTURY

Additional books and e-books in this series can be found on Nova's website under the Series tab.

PUBLIC HEALTH IN THE 21ST CENTURY

MORE PRESCRIPTION FOR CHANGE

CASE STUDIES FOR APPLICATIONS OF STRATEGY AND STRATEGIC INTERVENTION IN NATIONAL AND INTERNATIONAL HEALTH SYSTEMS IN RESPONSE TO A COVID PANDEMIC

LAURE PAQUETTE, PHD

nova
science publishers
New York

Library of Congress Cataloging-in-Publication Data

ISBN: 978-1-53619-097-7

Published by Nova Science Publishers, Inc. † New York

À la mémoire de Thelma Marion, sscj.

CONTENTS

Chapter 1

RAISING THE QUESTION

The goal of this book is to illustrate the uses of strategy in highly structured environments, both national and international. The case studies selected here are significant at the time of this writing: health care systems dealing with a COVID-19 pandemic. In systems, what is critical is the creativity of the strategist since the *marge de manoeuvre* is limited. In situations such as the COVID-19 pandemic, with its high degree of uncertainty, strategic intervention is particularly useful. The fundamentals of strategy, however, expounded over several previous books, continue to apply.

Readers familiar with my previous work know by now that I have taken an integrated approach to research on strategy along three axes. The first is a sequence of theoretical works exploring the concept of strategy as it applies to volitional actors, of which there are five types: individuals, infranational groups, supranational groups, states, and groups of states. The second axis is a series of illustrative case studies for each of those types of actors. Some of the cases are historical and some, as in the present work, are fictionalized. The third axis explores the various applications of strategy for these actors. Among the work already completed, for example, are how individuals and small groups can use strategy, how strategy can analyze national and international policy, and how strategy can analyze events of international significance.

For the Serious but not the Specialized Audience

Every professor employed by a university is expected to be productive: the question is what kind of production. Scholars as a group must develop critical methods to demonstrate their competence in a particular subject by what are primarily academic exercises. But the same can be said of scholars whose underlying consensus of attitude allow a unified comprehension of the subject, despite plenty of surface disagreements. It is to satisfy this aspiration that the present work addresses itself less to a purely academic audience than to a non-specialized public. This aspiration risks what Northrop Frye has experienced, with decisions that "confused even sympathetic academic reviewers, as well as driving others into all the hysterias of pedantry."[1]

Other reasons dictate my choice of format. One is a conviction that it is difficult to synthesize seemingly unrelated ideas into the sort of powerful theory that could genuinely explain the world and seek to change it. The second is this synthesis across disciplines and scholarly traditions is the answer to many of our problems in scholarship and, indeed, in our society. I have reached these conclusions after some thirty years' experience teaching and research: students can be introduced early to the most sophisticated of our various disciplinary theories and within a few weeks, be driving trucks through the gaps in them. I have a real concern over the importance of the realm of the mind in a post-COVID world. With the advent of more information rather than too little, it is likely that our powers of analysis are suffering attrition, compounded as they are by the vagaries of a scientism run rampant. With the crossover format attempted in these pages, I seek to leap those barriers and address myself to those who can use their

---

[1] Northrop Frye, *Words with Power* (New York: Harcourt Brace Jovanovich, 1990), xix-xx.

imaginations to pursue a better world, and who are not afraid to consider their actions as endowed with the significance that they undoubtedly have.

WHY FICTIONAL CASE STUDIES?

The book you are reading illustrates the use of strategy by national and international groups using fictional case studies. The cases are fictional in the sense that the information provided was not collected using the methodology used for my previous case studies about states or groups of states. I have instead combined characteristics and information as I saw necessary to make the example clear to the reader. The case studies presented reflect the categories outlined above: an infranational group strategizing to cope with a phenomenon, an individual, another infranational group, a supranational group, a government or state, and a group of government or states. It also includes the study of a phenomenon, here COVID-19. The case studies also meet certain structural requirements, having to illustrate each of the concepts (tactics, strategy) as well as the components of these concepts (core idea, goal). They show successful strategies that are not necessarily perfect. They show the fumbles as well as the lightning strikes.

The present book also differs from previous case studies to the extent that the various components of the strategy are not clearly identified. This will allow the self-taught strategist to use them to test their own skills at strategic analysis. The reason for this is simple: strategy is hard. It requires the reader to step back and see the big picture, when just about every other experience trained the reader to focus on the details. Even once the reader can set a clear goal, 90% of the energy goes to observing even the smallest changes in the strategy's environment, assessing which matter. Often the most experienced strategist will still have to choose between what is easy, what is fun, what is satisfying, and what will work. The smallest mistake can make the entire sequence of action collapse, even after months of work. There are no second chances, though there are always more opportunities. It is difficult to be hard-nosed about decisions, and yet it is critical for strategists not to delude themselves. A strategist routinely deals with situations about which information is limited, but without knowing to what extent. It is important to be analytical about the circumstances of a strategy and realistic about the chances of success, and yet equally important to be creative about core ideas. Discouraged yet? Think of the underdog, the one without power or money: for that person, strategy remains the best chance of achieving a goal.

FICTIONALIZED SETTING

Freedonia, featured in the 1933 Marx Brothers satirical film *Duck Soup*, is the setting for the case studies. It is a fictional state, a federation whose central government is responsible for delivering comprehensive health care. This health care system has a variety of problems, but it is now in crisis because its costs are now beyond what politicians are willing to pay. Politicians' concerns traditionally center on their own careers and re-election; as a result, they are sensitive to public opinion. In recent years, public opinion has evolved significantly: Freedonians no longer want governments to run big deficits, but neither do they want their taxes to increase or their services to be cut. Given these contradictions, politicians face a dilemma: so far, provincial governments have coped by pressing for more funds from the federal government, meanwhile trying to control costs.

Adding to the challenge are demographic trends. So-called baby-boomers are the most important bloc of voters in Freedonia: research shows that they expect to benefit from the latest research and technology, just as they reach the age where they will be using the health care system more and more. The tax base has been shrinking, and its rate of decline in real terms is expected to accelerate. Politicians have been generous to research supporting their positions. Most health services research looks at cost control or consequences of cost control: physician remuneration, impact of waiting lists, cost effectiveness of administration/delivery of services, and impact of service cuts. Cynics would say that the goal of much of this research is to avoid negative consequences or limit unintended ones. Essentially, research has focused on small-scale changes to the system. Incremental decision-making, however, will not be enough to meet the challenges.

State ministers of health announced a year ago that they would go ahead with radical reforms, over the federal government's objections if necessary. (The central government, aware of the problems from its vantage point, has been suggesting radical reform for some time.) Rufus T. Firefly, a former state politician, was appointed as sole commissioner for a Report on the Future of Health Care in Freedonia. His interim report argued that the time for radical change has arrived. The research community, meanwhile, tended to take a step back and consider the broader context, either theoretically or statistically. So far, there has been significant high-quality research in population studies. However, two of population health's limitations are: (1) it is not useful for solving system-wide problems; and (2) statistics necessarily strip away context. The ideal solution would be a process guiding decisions in managing and controlling change capable of considering the broader context and the trends. If all stakeholders had access to such a process, then not only could policy-makers make better decisions about reform, but health administrators could better manage and control the changes at their level, and clinicians and consumers better participate in planning and implementation. While there is such a process in international and domestic politics – strategy – there is no such process yet in the health field.

A few comments about the various Freedonian actors are in order. The regulated professions vary from province to province but they include: physiotherapists, nurses, physicians, dentists, optometrists, chiropractors, chiropodists, denture therapists, dental hygienists, radio technologists, audiologists, speech pathologists, dieticians, medical laboratory technicians, medical radiation technicians, midwives, respiratory therapists, massage therapists, psychologists, and pharmacists. For the purposes of this book, service providers also include analysts and researchers such as epidemiologists and academics. Stakeholders are usually understood to be patients and/or citizens. In the case of the provincial governments, all residents eligible for health care are stakeholders. Local managers include hospital and clinic administrators, as well as regional planners. Decision-makers include elected officials sitting on the executive of the federal or provincial governments and the people working to support those decisions and apply them. In Freedonia, the health care system has four levels: local, at which in most cases services are dispensed; regional for the purposes of planning of more specialized health services and decision-making; provincial for the administration of the health care system in that province; and federal, for certain types of decisions and policies, including some level of funding. There is also an international level, mostly at the level of research and exchange of information, sometimes for coordination for universal health concerns.

According to the typology of actors used for the purposes of strategic analysis, the infranational groups would include provincial non-governmental organizations (NGO's), provincial unions, professional associations, policy-makers, health administrators, patient groups, advocacy groups, and provincial companies. If we look at a provincial health care system as a system, then the supranational groups would be the national professional associations, the nation unions, the national policy makers, the national patient groups, companies, researchers, and NGO's. The states would include the provincial, the territorial and the municipal, whereas the groups of governments would be, for example, Freedonia, the European Union, the United States, Germany, and in general all countries that are federal.

METHOD

The method of construction of these case studies is one of composition and *gedankenexperimenten*, thought experiments, the technique pioneered by Albert Einstein in his development of his theory of relativity.[2] *Gedankenexperimenten* occur in the scientist' imagination so that they may

[2] N. Miscevic, (1992) "Mental Models and Thought Experiments", *International Studies in the Philosophy of Science*, 6:3, 215-226; J. Norton, "Are Thought Experiments Just What You Always Thought?" *Canadian Journal of Philosophy* (1996). I presume Stephen Hawking has proceeded in this manner, given his physical disabilities, but he does not refer to it explicitly.

investigate the effects of changes in concepts or conceptual details on theory rather than on reality.

Traditionally, scholarship has required the exposition of the method of development, so that readers may judge for themselves whether the conclusions reached are reliable. The process which has led to the framework of strategic analysis here includes six steps, shown in Table 1.1, Methodological Steps.

Table 1.1. Methodological Steps

Definition	Identify primary, secondary and methodological terms. Delineate, express essence Review using Aristotelian criteria
Brainstorm	Produce flood of suggestions, statements and relationships
Distillation	Break complex/compound statements down Differentiate by type Check accuracy Choose central statements
Ordering	Create set of statements by Ordering by type Establishing genealogy
Backward test	Check completion and parsimony
Operationalization	Make hypothesis observable operation Apply to a case

The definitions of the four key ideas for the purposes of this book are given in Table 1.2, Key Conceptual Definitions.

Values interact, strategies interact, and components of strategy interact. Those interactions can be neutral, identical, synergistic, cooperative, complementary, competitive, or antithetical (see Table 1.3, Possibilities of Strategic Interactions). Those interactions can also occur in varying degrees of intensity.

Table 1.2. Key Conceptual Definitions

Values	Heritage and most important standards cherished by individuals or groups
Decision	Process by which an actor selects a particular option out of many, designed to solve a particular problem[3]
Strategy	Imaginative idea which orchestrates and/or inspires sets of actions (tactics) in response to a given situation
Actor	Person or persons capable of action and decision; may be a state, non-governmental organization, or group

Table 1.3. Possibilities for Strategic Interactions

Possibility	Description
Neutrality	Strategies do not affect each other
Identity	2 strategies are identical
Synergy	When one national strategy reinforces the other
Cooperation	Deliberate, conscious common strategy addressing mutual concern
Complementarity	2 strategies address different concerns but in harmony with each other
Antithesis	two strategies in conflict

Any of the components of strategy (goals, tactics, core ideas) can interact, and any of these interactions can range among the possibilities outlined above. It is easy to imagine complementary interactions if one country's goals are direct and the other indirect, if one system's tactics are material and the other non-material, etc. For other components, like the core idea, the components are so central or so basic to the nature of the strategy

[3] Zeev Maoz, *National Choices and International Processes* (Cambridge: Cambridge University Press, 1989), 38. From a technical standpoint, the theory ought to refer to "choice", because it only addresses the middle step of policy. But in this case, "decision" and "decision-making" enjoy too great a currency for it to be practical to replace them. See Peter Carnevale and Rebecca A. Henry, "Determinants of Mediator Behaviour: A Test of the Strategic Choice Model," *Journal of Applied Social Psychology* 19:6 (1989), 481-498; John Friend and Allen Hickling, *Planning Under Pressure: The Strategic Choice Approach* (New York: Pergamon Press, 1987). The literature on strategic decision-making is sparse: Peter Linnert, *La stratégie militaire de Clausewitz et le management* (Trans. J.D. Hanaeur, Paris: Hommes et Techniques, 1972). It relies on a predetermined series of steps leading to a relatively correct conclusion, using inductive reasoning and creativity.

that any significant positive interaction necessitates the strategies being mutually known and mutually understood. Problems arise when they are not. The type of interaction may change if the strategy of one organization changes. The type of interaction may also change if any of the components of the strategy change.

Certain components change less frequently than others: values do not change frequently, for instance, but tactics can and do. The duration of various types of interactions, therefore, depends on the durability of the strategic components (see Table 1.4 Compatibility in the Short and Long-Term). Long-term compatibility means that there will be a lasting foundation for good relations.

Table 1.4. Compatibility in the Short and Long-Term

Component	Duration of Incompatibility
Strategy	Long
Values	Long
core idea	Medium
Goals	Short
Tactics	short

Compatibility exists when the two strategies are identical, neutral, cooperative, complementary, or synergistic at the global and the component level. Some components' interactions are more important than others, just as compatibility of certain components is essential to the compatible interactions of strategies. If the values are incompatible, however, then relations between actors are quite likely to be conflictual. It will also be more difficult to mobilize the population, in the case of liberal democracies at least, to accomplish the strategy.

SUBJECT AND STRUCTURE

There are various types of strategy, and the most common type of strategy is the strategy of the strong. *Inter alia*, however, it is underdog strategy that is discussed and promoted. Underdog strategy is the way of thinking of the weak and vanquished. The weak think differently from the strong, and it is hard for all members of society to start including those differences, if only because Aristotle deliberately excluded from future philosophical discourse the *mètis.*[4] Although this way of thinking did not disappear, consideration of it did, especially after the Aristotelian revival of the Renaissance.[5]

After the next two chapters introduce the theoretical foundations of strategy and strategic intervention, we move to the case studies. Chapter 9 provides a summary of the conclusions reached for the case studies and discusses the future research agenda.

---

[4] Marcel Detienne, *Les ruses de l'intelligence* (Paris: Flammarion, 1993), 124.

[5] Although daring, attempting such a correction is not without recent precedent. Philippe Nemo, *What Is the West?* (New York: Duquesne University Press, 2007).

Chapter 2

Strategic Development and Analysis

The theory used throughout these pages begins with the recognition that countries, governments, organizations, and individuals all have implicit or explicit objectives they wish to achieve. Success in reaching objectives may be fortuitous, but for consistently high-performing strategists, a core idea or slogan, which simplifies the complex goal they hope to achieve, is essential. Strategists must also design tactics by which their goal can be achieved.

A Novel Approach: Strategy in Health Care Systems

The idea of strategy has been occasionally applied to health care, usually in strategic planning and management. There have been some theoretical difficulties, and problems in proper implementation. The single most common problem has been for stakeholders to operate at a tactical, rather than a strategic, level. For several theoretical and epistemological reasons, the level of abstract thought needed for strategy is difficult to teach, and so it is difficult to plan and manage at a genuinely strategic level. Usually, strategic plans are detailed ways of controlling actions – in other words, tactical plans rather than strategic. When that is the case, strategic plans become irrelevant at circumstances change.

A review of the literature throws up both methodological and conceptual precedents for the application of strategy to the health system. Journal articles on clinical interventions use the word 'strategy' where, by the definitions given above, we would use the word 'tactics'.[6] These articles describe the success and impact that a series of actions have on particular illnesses or conditions. Journal articles on planning and management of health services or organizations either propose the use of a particular technique or report on its use in specific situations.[7] Chapters in books on health administration usually provide an overview of the different techniques or approaches available to the average hospital or clinic manager. [8] Both of these categories of publications share the business and management definition of strategy. By the definitions used in the coming pages, they are confusing strategy and tactics. This confusion does affect significant consequences for their uses: it makes successful strategic planning unlikely. Successful use of strategic planning and management is unusual. Strategic planning is effective in supporting the integration of health services, but "often falls prey to the unplanned external or internal forces at work in health care."[9] For strategy to be effective, there has to be very strong commitment from the decision-makers and a significant amount of time and energy from the rest of the organization: strategy is a drain on scarce resources, rather than the sometimes very noticeable catalyst in

---

6. Like V. Schmitz, C. Qian, J. Ruiz, B. Sangro, I. Melero, G. Mazzolini, I. Narvaiza and J. Prieto, "Gene Therapy for Liver Diseases: Recent Strategies for Treatment of Viral Hepatitis and Liver Malignancies," *Gut* 50:1 (January 2002):130-5.

7 Like A. R. Cox, "The art of strategic planning. Creating the future path", *AAOHN Journal.* 4:6(June 2001), 280-5, among many other examples.

8 Lawrence F. Wolper, *Health Care Administration/Planning, Implementing and Managing Organized Delivery Systems* (Gaithersburg, Maryland: Aspen, 1999, 3rd. ed.), 125; Roice D. Luke, James W. Begun and Steven Walston, "Strategy Making in Health Care Organizations," in Stephen M. Shortell and Arnold D. Kaluzny, *Health Care Management/ Organization Design and Behavior* (New York: Thomson, 1999, 4th Ed.), 394-431.

9 S. Glouberman and H. Mintzberg, "Managing the Care of Health and the Cure of Disease – Part II: Integration," *Health Care Management Review* 26:1 (Winter 2001), 70-84.D. Davidson, "Strategic Planning Myth or Reality", *Seminars for Nurse Managers* 8:2 (June 2000), 66-9, 6.

political or economic systems. The only examples of a similar definition being used are found in studies examining how academic medical centers try to use their clout and credibility when in conflict with their respective universities.[10]

Overall, the most important precedent for the use of strategy in health is the development of a completely new model for quality assurance, including applications in actual health organizations, over a ten-year period. In 1988, the European Foundation for Quality Management (EFQM) developed a self-assessment instrument on all levels of a health care organization, based on a new theoretical framework that was brought from the drawing board to the clinician's office in ten years. It is now used in the European Union as a framework for quality management, as a conceptualization for organizational excellence, as a guide for improvement projects, and as standards for the peer review of professional practices, accreditation, and certification.[11] Although the range of issues it addresses is narrower, the EFQM is more ambitious in application, since it had to develop all of its own theory, methodology, and training protocols.

What is proposed here, then, builds on previously established theory, method, and process. Strategy can enhance existing approaches to informing the decision-making process by restoring the context to models and analytical approaches, which otherwise strip research of contextual issues and their relevance to the complex pathways of health and empirical findings of population.[12] Strategy also offers a vehicle for bringing society's preferences, even when not rational, into the decision-making process, for balancing uncertainty and certainty, and for balancing complexity and simplicity.[13]

---

[10] W. W. Souba, M. R. Weitekamp and J. F. Mahon, "Political Strategy, Business Strategy and the Academic Medical Center: Linking Theory and Practice", *Journal of Surgical Research* 100:1 (September 2001), 1-10.

[11] U. Nabitz, N. Klazinga, J. Waslburg, "The EFQM Excellence Model: European and Dutch Experiences with the EFQM Approach in Health Care," *International Journal for Quality in Health care* 12:3 (June 2000): 191-201.

[12] S. Birch, "As a Matter of Fact: Evidence-Based Decision Making Unplugged," *Health Economics* 6:6 (November-December 1997), 547-59.

[13] J. Lynn and D. DeGrazia, "An Outcomes Model of Medical Decision Making," *Theoretical Medicine* 12:4 (December 1991), 325-43; D. W. Fraser, "Overlooked Opportunities for

The central hypothesis is that strategy and its related methods and tools can be adapted to manage and control change in a health care system, even in emergent situations such as COVID-19. The secondary hypotheses apply to the various levels and various types of stakeholders, e.g., stakeholders (patients, clinicians, health administrators, policy-makers) at each level (local, regional, national, international) can manage and control change in the health care system by using strategy and strategic thinking. Values are the independent variable: they are the heritage and most important standards cherished by the individual or society. Strategy and its components are the dependent variables. These components are: the goal (the aims or ends to which efforts are directed); the core idea (a central idea, usually a metaphor, which helps orchestrate actions); and the tactics (actions and resources useful or helpful to a desired end).

Strategy Step by Step

The present chapter also explains how to choose the basic components of strategy and then how to develop a strategy, step by step. This chapter also provides a sample of core ideas to either adopt within a strategy or to use to stimulate strategic thinking. By the end of this chapter, it will be possible to select the components of a strategy, choose a particular strategy, and generate a core idea. It is therefore essential to address the most common problem for strategists: distinguishing between strategy and tactics.

The knowledge transfer approach, called the worksheet system, assists in the development of a strategy, as opposed to the worksheets in the next chapter, whose goal is to develop a strategic intervention. The goal of the worksheets is not to provide an exhaustive set of described steps to reach a single correct conclusion. Rather, the intention here is to provide support for the art of designing or analyzing a strategy. In most cases, there are no single correct answers or correct ways to interpret the forms, and it is with

---

Investing in Health Research and Development," *Bulletin of the World Health Organization* 78:8 (January 2000): 1054-61.

trepidation that these instructions are even provided, since what matters is the engagement of the individual or group filling these out, not identifying a foolproof way of getting the right answer. The worksheets are not necessarily obvious to use at first, and to achieve conscious competence, the user needs to practice on average six or seven times. Once the user is proficient, however, s/he should only use the worksheets when there is a problem to be solved or as long as it is necessary for the strategy or strategic analysis to be completed in his/her mind.

The nine worksheets for the development of strategy are:

1. Strategy
2. Key Actors
3. An Actor's Actions or Tactics
4. Resources A Strategy Can Draw On
5. What You Can and Cannot Do
6. Factors Outside Your Control
7. Steps and Nodes
8. Tactics and Counter Tactics
9. Core idea.

Let us now consider the response to COVID-19 by the fictional Freedonian government. Freedonia's government is trying to minimize the number of people becoming infected or sick with COVID-19; minimize how sick people become; lower the mortality rate; manage the demand on the health care system; and help the population to manage risk. The response to COVID-19 has been informed by modelling of the impact of COVID-19. The modelling finds the health system will cope if Freedonia continues to have effective physical distancing, increase its health system capacity, and isolates people with the virus and their close contacts.

The Freedonian Health Protection Committee (FHPC) makes key decisions and coordinates this response. The FHPC is made up of the Chief Health Officers from each region, the Chief Medical Officer of Freedonia, and representatives from key departments. Freedonia is working with its partners in the health care system implementing a robust plan to monitor for, detect and, if needed, isolate any cases of the 2019 novel coronavirus. The Ministry of Health is taking several steps to ensure the health and safety of Freedonians. This includes:

- Enacting a declaration of emergency to help stop the spread and keep people safe.
- Monitoring hospitals for potential cases of the virus in individuals with travel history to areas under a travel health advisory for COVID-19.
- Adding the 2019 novel coronavirus as a designated disease reportable under Freedonia's public health legislation, enabling local public health units to quickly and effectively take all necessary measures to investigate, complete lab tests and do case and contact management to prevent and control further spread of the infection.
- Ongoing planning with regional partners and readiness to coordinate with other regions so they are prepared to respond quickly and effectively to any scenario, including: enhanced access to screening, expanding lab-testing capacity; and implementing new initiatives to keep the public and frontline workers safe.

Freedonia's Ministry of Health instructed public health care professionals to:

- Familiarize themselves with the interim national case definition for COVID-19 to consider the possibility of COVID-19 in persons with relevant clinical and exposure history.
- Familiarize themselves with the Interim National COVID-19 Case Report Form, to facilitate case reporting of confirmed and probable COVID-19 cases.
- Report confirmed and probable COVID-19 cases to FHPC within 24 hours of their own notification.
- Observe the Protocol for Microbiological Investigations of Severe Acute Respiratory Infections (SARI) to facilitate the diagnosis of severe respiratory infections due to both unknown and known

respiratory pathogens that have the potential for large-scale epidemics.

- Familiarize themselves with the guidance on the public health management of cases and contacts associated with COVID-19.

The COVID-19 pandemic has created unprecedented demand for certain supplies, including personal protective equipment (PPE). The government of Freedonia is using a range of strategies to respond to this increased demand by purchasing as many additional supplies as possible, increasing domestic production, and extending the use of N95 respirators through reprocessing, as required. Health Freedonia is closely tracking all potential drugs and vaccines in development in Freedonia and abroad. It is working with companies, academic research centers and investigators to help expedite the development and availability of treatments to prevent and treat COVID-19. Health Freedonia will prioritize the review of market authorization applications to facilitate earlier access to COVID-19 drugs or vaccines. It may also authorize access to the Freedonian market with certain restrictions. To support and expedite the authorization of drugs and vaccines for COVID-19 in Freedonia, the government is also collaborating with international counterparts and leveraging all available knowledge.

As the government learns more about COVID-19, it is regularly reviewing the response, moving resources into activities that are working well, and scaling back activities that are not working. The plan focuses on government activities. But many government and private agencies are working together to support the Freedonian government response. To reduce the risk of COVID-19 spreading through international travel, the government is applying travel restrictions, screening travelers who arrive in Freedonia and ensuring they quarantine on arrival and continuing with border surveillance.

Regional health authorities are testing people suspected of having the virus, monitoring close contacts of confirmed cases every day, imposing travel restrictions between regions, and opening fever clinics. The government urges the population to help stop the spread of the virus by:

- Staying informed through our COVID-19 health alert, which is updated every day.
- Keeping in touch with friends and family to make sure they are well.
- Taking steps to protect themselves and others, such as practicing good hygiene and quarantining themselves if they are sick.
- Staying healthy and making use of the ongoing support available; and
- Being a smart traveler — read the COVID-19 advice for travelers The government is also:
- Delivering a financial health package to protect all Freedonians.
- Expanding subsidized telehealth services for all Freedonians so everyone has access to quality healthcare while at home.
- Delivering support to Freedonians experiencing domestic, family, and sexual violence due to the fallout of coronavirus.
- Providing funds to support the mental health and wellbeing of Freedonians.
- Tracing coronavirus cases.
- Providing information on its response and how people can protect themselves and others in English and other languages; and
- Putting limits on some prescription and over the counter medications, to make sure those who need them can access them.

We can now explain the use of worksheets using Freedonia as an example.

Worksheet 1: Strategy

In this worksheet, the participant is expected to identify the components of a strategy to answer a particular challenge. The participant should use point form and no more than a single sheet to complete the worksheet. This will force him/her to be conceptually specific, and to choose among competing priorities. This way, it is possible to assess the judgment of the participant as well as his or her capacity to think using strategy.

Worksheet 1. Strategy		
Issue/Problem	COVID-19 Pandemic	
Goal	Reduce mortality	
Core idea (metaphor, slogan, etc.)	Bend the curve	
Tactics (actions or bundles of actions)	1	Minimize number of infected or ill people
	2	Minimize mortality rate
	3	Help population manage risk
	4	Manage demand on health care system

Those components are: the problem, to be described succinctly in the top box, "Issue"; the solution to that problem that suits the participant best, again to be described succinctly in the middle box, "Goal"; and the steps that will have the participant reach the goal, or the method he plans to use, of the collection of actions s/he plans to use, in the bottom box, "Tactics". A strategy need not be developed only in adversarial circumstances - it can be used to rise to a challenge of any type. But because it is demanding to develop and implement, it is usually only used in difficult or challenging circumstances where there are at least one and usually many enemy players. As usual, the participant must be detailed, specific, succinct, and must stay at one level of generality or detail throughout the worksheet.

WORKSHEET 2: KEY ACTORS

In any strategy, there are several, sometimes many, possible actors. Those actors can be individuals, groups, governments or even groups of governments. The actors can be involved in the planning of their own strategy or be on the outside. They may be helpful to a strategy, neutral, or opposed to it.

They may be conscious of strategy or actions, or they may not. But most importantly, they may have an impact either on the tactics or the strategy itself being analyzed, or designed, or carried out. The goal of this worksheet is to identify which ones may have an impact, so that the others can be set aside.

Worksheet 2. Key Actors	
All Actors	Can this actor affect your achieving the goal? (Yes or No)
Population	Y
Health care workers	Y
FHPC	Y
Chief health officer	Y
Regional chief health officers	Y
Representatives of key departments	Y
Ministry of Health	Y
Hospital administrators	Y
Local and regional public health units	Y
Local and regional labs units	Y
Frontline workers	Y
Public health care professionals	Y
Companies	Y
Academic research centers	Y
Academic investigators	Y
International counterparts	Y
Staff monitoring travelers	Y
People suffering mental health issues	Y
People suffering domestic, family, and sexual violence	Y
Pharmacists	Y

The specific instructions to complete this worksheet follow. For Column 1: give a comprehensive list of actors in the first column. List them under various headings, such as civilian, military, domestic, foreign, army, navy, air force, etc. Putting people or groups in the correct categories does not matter. Listing every individual and/or group possible does. Ask whether the groups listed ought to be broken down further into smaller groups.

For example, should a coalition of rape crisis centers be listed as such, or should it be broken down into the different member organizations? Once the comprehensive list of actors is established, the next column helps differentiate between significant and insignificant actors. In Column 2, ask: can this actor affect whether the tactic required can move the strategy toward the achievement of the goal. Ask whether can this actor affect achieving a goal? Or are there actors who stand no chance of affecting the outcome?

In the case of the Freedonian public health response, Worksheet 2 can be filled out in the above table.

Worksheet 3: An Actor's Actions and Tactics

The next step in the tactical analysis of a situation focuses on the tactics, and similarly differentiates significant from insignificant actions, using Worksheet 3: An Actor's Actions and Tactics. There are several actions on the part of each significant actor. Those actions may be tactics, i.e., relevant to the strategy, or not. To be tactics, they must directly or indirectly move the situation towards the goal being achieved. Tactics themselves may prevent the goal from being achieved or the strategy from being successful, i.e., they can be key tactics.

The specific instructions to complete this worksheet follow. For Column 1: give the date and time of the action being analyzed. During the first draft, list actions as remembered, but in later draft it is helpful to list them chronologically. Only if more than one action takes place on a particular day is the time listed. For Column 2: give a detailed description of the action you are considering. Use point form rather than full sentences: this will help focus on the most important features of the action. For Column 3: an action is a tactic if it is relevant to the achievement of the goal identified in the strategy. If the answer to the question: "Does this affect reaching my goal in any way?" If the answer is yes, then the action is a tactic.

Worksheet 3. An Actor's Actions		
Actor: Government		
Time/Date	Action	Is this a tactic? (Yes/No)
Not given	Models of the impact of COVID-19	Y
Not given	Assigns FHPC power to make key decisions and coordinate response	Y
Not given	Declares emergency	Y
Not given	Monitors hospitals for potential cases of the virus in travelers	Y
Not given	Adds the 2019 novel coronavirus as reportable disease	Y
Not given	Readies for coordination with other regions	Y
Not given	Plans with regional partners	Y
Not given	Instructs public health care professionals on COVID policy and procedures	Y
Not given	Works to respond to increased demand for certain supplies	Y
Not given	Reviews its response regularly	Y
Not given	Applies travel restrictions	Y
Not given	Instructs population on how to help stop spread of virus	Y
Not given	Delivers a financial health package to protect all Freedonians	Y
Not given	Expands subsidized telehealth services	Y
Not given	Supports Freedonians experiencing domestic, family, and sexual violence due to the fallout of coronavirus	Y
Not given	Funds mental health services	Y
Not given	Traces coronavirus cases	Y
Not given	Provides information on how the population can protect itself	Y
Not given	Puts limits on some prescription and over the counter medications	Y

Worksheet 4: Resources a Strategy Can Draw On

The third step is the identification of resources, using Worksheet 4: Resources a Strategy Can Draw On. Put at its broadest, resources which make tactics possible are generated by "the symbolic experiences, mythic lore, and ritual practices of a group or society [that] create moods and motivations, ways of organizing experience and evaluating reality, modes of regulating conduct, and way of forming social bonds."[14] Conventional wisdom usually finds that money is the most important resource, and it can certainly be a severely limiting factor. Much more scarce and harder to increase, however, is the attention and good will of people with power. It is also much easier to squander inadvertently. The four general types of resources discussed below are: the right equipment, the right people, time, and information.

Although more ink is spilled and meetings held on money and money-related issues than anything else, the most important resource is human: skills, energy, and number. The first step is to establish what skills are useful, and then scan for them among the significant actors. Among the non-technical skills that may be needed are counseling, writing, speaking, planning, research, tactical analysis, strategic analysis, forecasting, calm under pressure, good judgment, integrity. Worksheet 4: Resources A Strategy Can Draw On should be filled out listing as many of the resources as possible.

The specific instructions to complete this worksheet follow. For Column 1: List here all the materials, services, people (beyond the people who are carrying out the strategy with you), information, and funds that needed to achieve the goal. The list should be comprehensive, i.e., it should include absolutely everything you will need. To increase the chances of writing a comprehensive list, it is helpful to look at categories of resources, so that resources are less likely to be forgotten anything. Categories include at least goods, services, people, information, and funds. It is also possible to develop categories that are specific to a situation, as has been done in sample Worksheet 4.

For Column 2: answer here the question of whether there is enough of this resource for you to reach the goal. For example, if the collective is considering extending its hours of operations, it may incur extra expenses, or need to hire more people. Is more money available, and if so, is it on a one-time or long-term basis? Even if there is enough for foreseeable needs,

---

[14] Ann Swidler, "Culture in Action: Symbols and Strategies," *American Sociological Review* 51:2 (April 1986), 273-286.

or even more than foreseeable needs, it is still a specific amount available. Whether the resource is limited or not is an important point for carrying out the strategy. The strategist needs to consider the limited resources as the strategy unfolds.

For Column 3: here, ask whether the resource being analyzed is necessary for reaching the goal, whether if there is none of this resource left the goal could still achieved. If so, then write 'yes' in this column. Whether the resource is limited or not is an important point for carrying out the strategy, but if it is an essential resource, then the strategist must put it at the highest priority. The list below is an illustration of the type of analysis that needs to be done; it is not a complete list of resources necessary.

For Column 4: Is the resource being analyzed helpful to the goal being reached? Is it something that will move the strategy forward? If so, the answer is yes. Only the 'yes' resources need to be analyzed further.

For the Freedonian public health response, Worksheet 4 can be completed as follows:

Worksheet 4. Resources			
	Do you have enough? (Yes/No)	Is this a 'nice to have?'	Is this a 'must have'?
Resource			
Information for modelling	N		Y
Time for modelling	Y		Y
Expertise for modelling	Y		Y
Money to pay for modelling	Y		Y
Information for FHPC	N		Y
Time for FHPC	N		Y
Money for FHPC	Y	Y	
Outside expertise for FHPC	Y	Y	
Time for working with health care system partners	N		Y
Money for working with health care system partners	N		Y
Expertise for working with health care system partners	Y		Y
Information for working with health care system partners	N		Y
Expertise for training public health professionals	Y		Y
Information for training public health professionals	N		Y
Money for training public health professionals	Y		Y
Time training public health professionals	N		Y

Worksheet 4. Resources			
	Do you have enough? (Yes/No)	Is this a 'nice to have?'	Is this a 'must have'?
Information for purchasing certain supplies	Y		Y
Money for purchasing certain supplies	Y		Y
Time for purchasing certain supplies	Y		Y
Information for manufacturing certain supplies	Y		Y
Money for manufacturing certain supplies	Y		Y
Time for manufacturing certain supplies	N		Y
Expertise for ongoing review of government response	Y		Y
Information for ongoing review of government response	Y		Y
Money for ongoing review of government response	Y		Y
Time for ongoing review of government response	Y		Y
Money for screening population	Y		Y
Information for screening population	N		Y
Expertise for screening population	Y		Y
Time for screening population	N		Y
Money for screening travelers	Y		Y
Information for screening travelers	Y		Y
Expertise for screening travelers	Y		Y
Time for screening travelers	Y		Y
Time to educate population	N		Y
Money to educate population	N		Y
Information to educate population	N		Y
Expertise to educate population	Y		Y
Time to monitor population	N		Y
Money to monitor population	N		Y
Information to monitor population	Y		Y
Expertise to monitor population	Y		Y
Money for financial health package for Freedonians	Y		y
Money for support on mental health	Y		Y
Expertise for support on mental health	Y		Y
Information for support on mental health	Y		Y
Information for support on domestic, family, or sexual violence	Y		Y
Expertise or support on domestic, family, or sexual violence	Y		Y
Money for support on domestic, family, or sexual violence	Y		Y

WORKSHEET 5: WHAT YOU CAN AND CANNOT DO

The fifth step in the tactical analysis requires an examination of the rules. Rules can be either formal or informal, and they may be incomplete; if dealing with hostiles, these rules may not be obvious. Rules are enforced through sanctions, so one way to spot informal systems is to watch for behavior changes among the hostile actors, and then look for the factors that led to the modification. Sanctions tend to be obvious.

The specific instructions to complete this worksheet follow.

For Column 1: List here all the formal and informal rules about materials, services, people (beyond the people who are carrying out the strategy), information, and funds that you need to achieve your goal. The list should be comprehensive, i.e., it should include absolutely everything needed. To increase the chances of writing a comprehensive list, it is helpful to look at categories of rules, listed above, making it less likely anything is forgotten. Categories are the same as for resources: goods and services, people, information, and funds. Categories may also be developed for a specific situation.

For Column 2: Is the rule being analyzed helpful to the goal being reached? Is it something that will move the strategy forward? If so, the answer is yes. For Column 3: here, ask if disregarding this rule will ensure the failure of the strategy. Rules constrain behavior, but it is important to be aware of how and why each rule constrains which behavior or action. Ask if the rule being analyzed is necessary for reaching the goal, whether if this rule is broken or ignored, whether the goal could still achieve. Answer 'yes' or 'no'. For those rules, the strategist must put it at the highest priority. The list below is an illustration of the type of analysis that needs to be done; it is not a complete list of rules necessary.

For the COVID-19 case study, this worksheet can be completed as follows:

Worksheet 5. What you can and cannot do		
Rule	Does this rule help you reach your goal?	Does breaking this rule guarantee your failure?
Laws on government spending	Y	N
Regulations on government spending	Y	N
Policies on government spending	Y	N
Procedures on government spending	Y	N
Professional ethics, health professions	Y	N
Collective agreements for front line workers	Y	N
Laws on social distancing	Y	Y
Regulations on social distancing	Y	Y
Policies on social distancing	Y	Y
Procedures on social distancing	Y	Y
Laws on tracing and isolation	Y	Y
Regulations on tracing and isolation	Y	Y
Policies on tracing and isolation	Y	Y
Procedures on tracing and isolation	Y	Y
Laws on hospitals and clinics	Y	N
Regulations on hospitals and clinics	Y	N
Policies on hospitals and clinics	Y	N
Procedures on hospitals and clinics	Y	N
State of emergency legislation	Y	Y
Laws on travel restrictions	Y	Y
Regulations on travel restrictions	Y	Y
Policies on travel restrictions	Y	Y
Procedures on travel restrictions	Y	Y
Laws on infectious diseases	Y	Y
Regulations on infectious diseases	Y	Y
Policies on infectious diseases	Y	Y
Procedures on infectious diseases	Y	Y
Laws on purchasing, distributing, and manufacturing PPE	Y	Y
Regulations on purchasing, distributing, and manufacturing PPE	Y	Y
Policies on purchasing, distributing, and manufacturing PPE	Y	Y
Procedures on purchasing, distributing, and manufacturing PPE	Y	Y
Protocol for Microbiological Investigations of Severe Acute Respiratory Infections (SARI)	Y	Y
Guidance on the public health management of cases and contacts	Y	Y
Laws on market authorization applications	Y	N

Worksheet 5. What you can and cannot do		
Rule	Does this rule help you reach your goal?	Does breaking this rule guarantee your failure?
Regulations on market authorization applications	Y	N
Policies on market authorization applications	Y	N
Procedures on market authorization applications	Y	N
Laws on prescription and over the counter medications	Y	N
Regulations on prescription and over the counter medications	Y	N
Policies on prescription and over the counter medications	Y	N
Procedures on prescription and over the counter medications	Y	N

Worksheet 6: Factors Outside Your Control

Factors are events, actions, trends, tactics outside any actors' control. For the Freedonian public health response, Worksheet 6 can be filled out in the following way:

Worksheet 6. Factors Outside Your Control			
Desired Strategic Outcome: reduced mortality and morbidity			
Factors that help		Factors that do not help	
	→	←	Natural disaster

The desired strategic outcome is the goal listed in the strategy. These may include goals drawn from a variety of categories. Factors that help may include public anxiety, political pressure, or pressure on other institutions of society. Factors that do not help situation may include budget constraints, lack of information, few effective measures, and lack of experience.

WORKSHEET 7: DO OR DIE MOMENTS

The strategic pathway is the succession of steps which are likeliest to lead to the achievement of the goal. It can be identified using a three-step process: first, all possible steps to the goal are identified; second, the significant steps out of all the possible ones are identified; third, the critical steps are identified. The strategic pathway is made up of the critical steps, i.e., strategic nodes. Worksheet 7: Do or Die Moments, asks the following questions: what are the steps to achieving the goal? For each step, what are the alternative steps that can also lead to goal? What are the scenarios that will achieve the goal? Who decides? Who has the power to make the changes? What are the other possibilities? Are any of the alternatives more effective? Are any more economical, not just in terms of money, but also in terms of other resources? Are any more likely to succeed? What arguments are convincing to those who decide? What factors affect the decisions of those who decide? Working backwards, how would the steps be listed? Worksheet 7 also assists in identifying the do-or-die moments. Among the questions are: what are the critical actors, actions, resources, rules? Where are they situated on in relationship to another? Is the strategy focused on the strategic nodes? Are efforts concentrated there? How does this change how to reach goals?

The specific instructions for filling out the worksheet follow. The strategic goal is the goal that is given in the strategy from worksheet 1. In the first column, write out each of the steps necessary to reach the goal, in sequence. This first column is for reaching the goal with no surprises or problems. Fill in the steps until you reach your goal. Each step should represent a single tactic or action contributing to your goal. List all the steps necessary to reach your goal.

Next, identify which steps are essential to reaching the goal. Consider each step and ask whether it would still be possible to reach the goal if the strategy failed at this step. If the answer is 'yes', then circle that step. That is a strategic node, and the strategy needs to have alternatives to make sure that it gets beyond that step. In the middle column, write alternative steps to reach the goal for each of the problems at a strategic node. If at any point the pathway starts to be the same as in column 1, then just draw an arrow returning to that step.

Next, identify which steps are essential to reaching the goal. Consider each step and ask whether it would still be possible to reach the goal if the current tactic listed failed. If the answer is 'yes', then circle that step. That is a strategic node: develop an alternative to make sure the strategy gets past it.

In the right-hand column, fill in the steps to reach the goal if another set of problems occurs after what the predictions in the middle column. Again, fill in the steps until the goal is reached, and if at any point the pathway starts to be the same as in the middle or left-hand column, then just draw an arrow returning to that step. Use more than one copy of the worksheet if necessary. Remember to number the worksheets sequentially if necessary.

For the Freedonian public health response, Worksheet 7 can be filled out in the following way:

Worksheet 7. Do or Die Moments		
Goal: reduce mortality and morbidity from COVID-19		
Problem 1	Problem 2	Problem 3
Models of the impact of COVID-19 ▼		
Assigns FHPC power to make key decisions and coordinate response ▼		
Declares emergency ▼		
Monitors hospitals for potential cases of the virus in travelers ▼		
Adds the 2019 novel coronavirus as reportable disease ▼		
Readies for coordination with other regions ▼		
Plans with regional partners ▼		
Instructs public health care professionals on COVID policy and procedures		

Worksheet 7. Do or Die Moments		
Goal: reduce mortality and morbidity from COVID-19		
Problem 1	Problem 2	Problem 3
▼		
Realizes the shortages of certain supplies	Works to respond to increased demand for certain supplies ▼	
	Reviews its response regularly ▼	
	Applies travel restrictions ▼	
	Instructs population on how to help stop spread of virus ▼	
	Realizes pandemic is creating several other major problems ▼	Delivers a financial health package to protect all Freedonians ▼
		Expands subsidized telehealth services ▼
		Supports Freedonians experiencing domestic, family, and sexual violence due to the fallout of coronavirus ▼
		Funds mental health services ▼
		Puts limits on some prescription and over the counter medications

WORKSHEET 8: TACTICS AND COUNTER TACTICS

Once the analysis is complete, choose tactics for their economy and maximum benefit. If that is not apparent, it is possible to develop multiple scenarios for outcomes, depending on how favorable various factors are to the tactic, using Worksheet 8: Tactics and Counter Tactics. Questions to ask in terms of this latest worksheet include: who decides? Who has the power to make the changes? What are the other possibilities? Are any of the alternatives more effective? Are they economical in terms of personnel, resources? Who is likely to succeed? What arguments are convincing to those who decide? What factors affect the decisions of those who decide? If you were to work backwards, how would you set the steps? For the next phase, start with steps, then actors, then factors, then resources, then actions/tactics, then at last rules for system analysis.

The specific instructions for filling out Worksheet 8 are as follows. The two columns represent the tactics of two actors. On the left list tactics, and on the right is another actor with a different goal. The goals need not be contradictory: they need only not be identical. Under the heading Tactics, on the left, list all the actions that move that actor towards the strategic goal chosen.

Worksheet 8. Tactics and Counter Tactics			
Your Goal:		Their Goal:	
Your Tactics		Their Countervailing Tactics	
	→	←	
	→	←	
	→	←	
	→	←	
	→	←	
	→	←	
	→	←	
	→	←	
	→	←	
	→	←	
	→	←	
	→	←	
	→	←	
	→	←	

Under the heading Countervailing Tactics, on the right, list all the actions that move that actor towards the other strategic goal chosen. The tactics and counter tactics do not have to match up, although many of them will. The list on each side needs to be complete, so that it may be useful to use categories again.

For the Freedonian public health response, Worksheet 8 need not be filled out since the virus is a phenomenon, not an actor.

WORKSHEET 9: CORE IDEA

Because coming up with a core idea is often the most difficult part of the exercise, here is a short worksheet that can be completed quickly to stimulate thinking about it. This worksheet is designed to force the thinking beyond the rational, linear model that has served so far so well. The goal of the worksheet is to get the process of thinking metaphorically established, and then to provide an opportunity for some practice. It is deliberately simple to foster and focus thinking with strategy. Not all the metaphors are practical or helpful. The point is to produce several, developing the capacity to judge which are better or more practical. The specific instructions for filling out Worksheet 9 follow.

In the third column, list the metaphors, images, role models or images that come to mind that fit the same category. In the fourth column, chose one image or metaphor and work it into a slogan that captures how the goal can be achieved. Repeat these steps for the other categories. At the bottom of the page is a blank space to write in a category of images and metaphors that come to mind. Then list the images or metaphors that come to mind, and develop a slogan using that metaphor or image.

For the Freedonian public health response, Worksheet 9 can be completed as follows:

Worksheet 9. Core idea			
Category	Suggested Metaphors, Images, Analogies, Role Models	Your Metaphors, Images, Role Models, Analogies	Core idea
Military	Machine gun, rifle, tank	submarine	Come to port unobserved
Geographical	River, waterfall, creek	Pond	Still waters run deep
Plant	Tree, fern, Venus flytrap	Roots	Root action in principles
Transportation	Bus, golf cart, car	Subway	Get to the point without getting bogged down in traffic

Worksheet 9. Core idea			
Category	Suggested Metaphors, Images, Analogies, Role Models	Your Metaphors, Images, Role Models, Analogies	Core idea
Sports	Caddy, gymnastics, football		
Mechanical	Wrench, Allen key, ratchet		
Insects	Mosquito, ant, butterfly		
Animals	Cougar, puma rhinoceros		
Role models	Princess Diana, Donald Trump, Gandhi		
Your own Category: geometry	Your own metaphors: shapes	Curve	Bend the curve

This chapter covered the basics of developing a strategy. The next chapter outlines the basics of a strategic intervention in a crisis.

Chapter 3

STRATEGIC INTERVENTION: MAKING THE BEST OF A BAD IDEA

Tactical analysis, for our purposes, is the analysis and prediction of another actor's behaviour. It is similar to the development or analysis of strategy since it is also a multi-step process, and it is based on the same fundamental distinctions between what matters and what does not – for actions, for actors, for resources, for rules, and for factors. However, strategic intervention is the design of tactics in a crisis, and it is therefore essential to ensure that they are distinguished clearly from strategy. Strategic intervention may not be intuitively obvious for all readers, and to assist them this chapter provides a second set of worksheets. The worksheets come with instructions as well as a first illustration with a case study, the same as in Chapter 2. And like the set presented in Chapter 2, readers may need to use the process three or four times before it becomes easier.

The first step in developing a strategic intervention is making sure that a strategic intervention is what is needed. Worksheet 10: Nature of the crisis is designed to identify whether a change of strategy is needed. It asks fundamental questions, such as whether the situation is so grave that you may have to choose among values to deal with it. If that is the case, then the worksheets in Chapter 2 are needed. However, if a change of tactics is sufficient, then it is possible to proceed to the next worksheet.

WORKSHEET 10: NATURE OF THE CRISIS

The lower the first yes occurs in the answer column, the less grave the crisis. If the answer is yes at 4 or above, you need to develop a new strategy. Otherwise, the strategic intervention can be designed. Strategic intervention is not about a new strategy, which is assumed to be sound, but about major adjustments to the strategy.

In the case of the Freedonian public health response, the decision is up to the government. This government must decide whether a strategic intervention is necessary.

Worksheet 10. Nature of the Crisis	
Question	Answer (Y/N)
1. Do you have to change the values?	N
Choices are: • Between self-orientation and communitarianism? • Between materialism and non-materialism?	 Communitarianism Non-materialism
2. Do you have to choose among the values for a priority?	Y
Choices are: • Self-orientations over materialism or non-materialism • Community orientation over materialism or non-materialism • Materialism over self orientation or community orientation • Non-materialism over self orientation or community orientation	 N N N Y
3. Do you have to change the type of strategy?	Y
Choices are: • To direct strategy of action • To direct strategy of persuasion • To indirect strategy of action • To indirect strategy of persuasion	 N N N Y
4. Do you have to change the core idea?	Y
5. Do you have to change the categories of tactics?	Y

Since it is now clear that a strategic intervention is necessary, then it is possible to proceed to Worksheet 11, Events Leading Up to the Crisis.

WORKSHEET 11: EVENTS LEADING UP TO THE CRISIS

The general instructions are as follows: in column 1, list events in chronological order as they occurred, until the first unplanned event. List the first unplanned event in column 2, and then list the actions taken to cope with this unplanned event, again in chronological order. List all the coping actions taken until it is possible to return to the plan, and then list those. At the second unplanned event, move to column 3 and list the unplanned event there, and then list the actions taken to cope with this unplanned event, in chronological order. Then list the events and actions once it was possible to return to the plan. Repeat this process until there is a list of all events to date.

Turning now to the response by the Freedonian government, we can posit the following.

Worksheet 11. Events Leading up to the Crisis					
Models of the impact of COVID-19					
Assigns FHPC power to make key decisions and coordinate response					
Declares emergency					
Monitors hospitals for potential cases of the virus in travelers					
Adds the 2019 novel coronavirus as reportable disease					
Readies for coordination with other regions					
Plans with regional partners					
Instructs public health care professionals on COVID policy and procedures					

If the situation is too complex to be represented on a single worksheet, analyze a single category of tactics for each worksheet, and repeat until the situation is completely mapped out.

Worksheet 12:
Tactics Before and During the Crisis

It is common for a strategy to have between three and five groups of tactics. These naturally would have been applied leading up to the crisis. The present worksheet is designed to identify at what point the tactics became affected by the crisis. As well, this table lists actions taken to cope with the crisis, so that any further action can be considered in context.

Worksheet 12. Tactics Before and During the Crisis		
Event	Type	Tactic

In the preceding worksheet, it was possible to break down the situation into its component actions. Only the actions know to the analyst are listed – this is normal in a real situation. Once that task is done, then it is possible to analyze from several points of view. In this next worksheet, it is possible to identify what tactics were used, and to distinguish those tactics from the actions occurring as part of the crisis. It means, among other things, that it is possible to assess the effectiveness of each set of tactics, and it is also possible to assess possible courses of actions. We can see the Freedonian government's crisis below. The contents in Column 1 of Worksheet 12 are drawn from the events listed in Worksheet 11.

Now that the analysis has been completed, the next step is to identify which actors can, in this crisis, affect the outcome.

The first thing to do is to cut and paste the tactics from the previous two worksheets into the next worksheet. It is best to prepare a worksheet per category of tactic. The first step is to identify possible key actors using Worksheet 13, Possible Key Actors.

Worksheet 12. Tactics Before and During the Crisis		
Event	Type	Tactic
Realizes the shortages of certain supplies	Crisis	1
Works to respond to increased demand for certain supplies	Coping	1
Realizes pandemic is creating several other major problems	Crisis	2
Delivers a financial health package to protect all Freedonians	Coping	2
Expands subsidized telehealth services	Coping	3
Supports Freedonians experiencing domestic, family, and sexual violence due to the fallout of coronavirus	Coping	4
Funds mental health services	Coping	5
Puts limits on some prescription and over the counter medications	Planned	1

WORKSHEET 13: POSSIBLE KEY ACTORS

Worksheet 13. Key Actors	
Number	Key Actors
1	Freedonian government
2	Ministry of Health
3	Chief Health Officer

WORKSHEET 14: KEY ACTORS BY TACTIC

Worksheet 14, Key Actors by Tactic, assists in this. In column one, lists all the actions taken within one group of tactics. Identify the five most significant actors, list their names in line 1, then answer whether this actor can affect the outcome of this particular action.

Worksheet 14. Key Actors by Tactic			
Category of Tactic: ______________________			
Tactic	Can Key Actor 1 Affect? (Y/N)	Can Key Actor 2 Affect? (Y/N)	Can Key Actor 3 Affect? (Y/N)

In the case of the Freedonian government, the worksheets are completed as follows.

Worksheet 14. Key Actors by Tactic			
Category of Tactic: ________crisis_______________			
Tactic	Can Key Actor 1 Affect? (Y/N)	Can Key Actor 2 Affect? (Y/N)	Can Key Actor 3 Affect? (Y/N)
Realizes the shortages of certain supplies	Y	Y	Y
Realizes pandemic is creating several other major problems	Y	Y	Y

Worksheet 14. Key Actors by Tactic			
Category of Tactic: ______coping_________________			
Tactic	Can Key Actor 1 Affect? (Y/N)	Can Key Actor 2 Affect? (Y/N)	Can Key Actor 3 Affect? (Y/N)
Works to respond to increased demand for certain supplies	Y	Y	N
Delivers a financial health package to protect all Freedonians	Y	N	N
Expands subsidized telehealth services	Y	Y	N
Supports Freedonians experiencing domestic, family, and sexual violence due to the fallout of coronavirus	Y	Y	N
Funds mental health services	Y	Y	N

Worksheet 14. Key Actors by Tactic			
Category of Tactic: ________planned_______________			
Tactic	Can Key Actor 1 Affect? (Y/N)	Can Key Actor 2 Affect? (Y/N)	Can Key Actor 3 Affect? (Y/N)
Puts limits on some prescription and over the counter medications	Y	Y	N

In this case, the tactics are relatively few. It is possible that repeating this worksheet for each category of tactic will be necessary. It is more usual to complete 4 or 5 of these.

Worksheet 15: Key Rules

Once the previous worksheets are completed, analyze the rules by group of tactics. The first step in analyzing the situation of the collective is to list the possible key rules, and the second is to duplicate the tactics by category. These are listed in Worksheet 15, Key Rules

Worksheet 15. Key Rules	
Number	Possible Key Rule
1	
2	
3	
4	

In the case of the Freedonian government, the worksheets are completed as follows.

Worksheet 15. Key Rules	
Number	Possible Key Rule
1	Laws on infectious diseases
2	Professional ethics for health professionals
3	Procedures on tracing and isolating
4	Collective agreements for front line workers

WORKSHEET 16: KEY RULES BY TACTIC

For Worksheet 16, Key Rules by Tactic, list in column one all the actions taken within one particular group of tactics. Identify the five most significant rules, list them in line 1, then answer whether this actor affect the outcome of this particular action. It is important to remember to include both formal and explicit rules, as well as informal or implicit rules. Repeat this worksheet for each category of tactic.

Worksheet 16. Key Rules by Tactic				
Category of Tactic: ____________________				
Tactic	Can Key Rule 1 Affect? (Y/N)	Can Key Rule 2 Affect? (Y/N)	Can Key Rule 3 Affect? (Y/N)	Can Key Rule 4 Affect? (Y/N)

For the Freedonian government, Worksheet 16 can be completed as follows.

Worksheet 16. Key Rules by Tactic				
Category of Tactic: ________crisis______________				
Tactic	Can Key Rule 1 Affect? (Y/N)	Can Key Rule 2 Affect? (Y/N)	Can Key Rule 3 Affect? (Y/N)	Can Key Rule 4 Affect? (Y/N)
Realizes the shortages of certain supplies	N	N	N	Y
Realizes pandemic is creating several other major problems	N	N	N	Y

Worksheet 16. Key Rules by Tactic				
Category of Tactic: ____________coping__________				
Tactic	Can Key Rule 1 Affect? (Y/N)	Can Key Rule 2 Affect? (Y/N)	Can Key Rule 3 Affect? (Y/N)	Can Key Rule 4 Affect? (Y/N)
Works to respond to increased demand for certain supplies	N	N	N	N
Delivers a financial health package to protect all Freedonians	N	N	N	Y
Expands subsidized telehealth services	N	N	N	N
Supports Freedonians experiencing domestic, family, and sexual violence due to the fallout of coronavirus	N	N	N	Y
Funds mental health services	N	N	N	Y

Worksheet 16. Key Rules by Tactic				
Category of Tactic: ______planned________________				
Tactic	Can Key Rule 1 Affect? (Y/N)	Can Key Rule 2 Affect? (Y/N)	Can Key Rule 3 Affect? (Y/N)	Can Key Rule 4 Affect? (Y/N)
Puts limits on some prescription and over the counter medications	N	Y	N	N

WORKSHEET 17: KEY RESOURCES

The first step in analyzing the situation of the Freedonian government is to list the possible key resources in Worksheet 17, and the second is to duplicate the tactics by category.

Worksheet 17. Key Resources	
Number	Possible Key Resource
1	
2	
3	
4	
5	

For Freedonia, it is possible to complete the worksheet as follows.

Worksheet 17. Key Resources	
Number	Possible Key Resource
1	Time for manufacturing certain supplies
2	Information for ongoing review of government response
3	Money for working with health care system partners
4	Information for training public health professionals
5	Expertise for screening population

It is now possible to complete Worksheet 18, Key Resources by Tactic. For this worksheet, in Column 1, lists all the actions taken within one group of tactics. Identify the five most significant resources, list their names in line 1, then ask whether this actor affect the outcome of this particular action. It is important to list resources in each of the four categories: money, time, information, and people. Repeat this worksheet for each category of tactic.

Worksheet 18. Key Resources by Tactic					
Category of Tactic: ____________________					
Tactic	Can Key Resource 1 Affect? (Y/N)	Can Key Rule 2 Affect? (Y/N)	Can Key Resource 3 Affect? (Y/N)	Can Key Resource 4 Affect? (Y/N)	Can Key Resource 5 Affect? (Y/N)

Freedonian authorities can fill out this worksheet as follows.

Worksheet 18. Key Resources by Tactic					
Category of Tactic: _____crisis__________________					
Tactic	Can Key Resource 1 Affect? (Y/N)	Can Key Rule 2 Affect? (Y/N)	Can Key Resource 3 Affect? (Y/N)	Can Key Resource 4 Affect? (Y/N)	Can Key Resource 5 Affect? (Y/N)
Realizes the shortages of certain supplies	N	Y	N	N	N
Realizes pandemic is creating several other major problems	N	Y	N	N	N

Worksheet 18. Key Resources by Tactic					
Category of Tactic: _____coping__________________					
Tactic	Can Key Resource 1 Affect? (Y/N)	Can Key Rule 2 Affect? (Y/N)	Can Key Resource 3 Affect? (Y/N)	Can Key Resource 4 Affect? (Y/N)	Can Key Resource 5 Affect? (Y/N)
Works to respond to increased demand for certain supplies	Y	Y	N	N	N
Delivers a financial health package to protect all Freedonians	N	Y	N	N	N
Expands subsidized telehealth services	N	Y	N	N	N
Supports Freedonians experiencing domestic, family, and sexual violence due to the fallout of coronavirus	N	Y	N	N	N
Funds mental health services	N	Y	Y	N	N

Worksheet 18. Key Resources by Tactic					
Category of Tactic: _______planned_________________					
Tactic	Can Key Resource 1 Affect? (Y/N)	Can Key Rule 2 Affect? (Y/N)	Can Key Resource 3 Affect? (Y/N)	Can Key Resource 4 Affect? (Y/N)	Can Key Resource 5 Affect? (Y/N)
Puts limits on some prescription and over the counter medications	N	Y	Y	N	N

Once completed, repeat the process for Worksheets 19, Possible Key Factors, and 20, Key Factors by Tactic. The first step in analyzing the situation of the collective is to list the possible key factors, in Worksheet 19, and the second is to duplicate the tactics by category.

WORKSHEET 19: POSSIBLE KEY FACTORS

For this worksheet, in column one, lists all the actions taken within one group of tactics. Then identify the five most significant Factors, list them in line 1, then ask whether this factor can affect the outcome of this particular action. It is important to list Factors in each of the four categories: money, time, information, and people. Repeat this worksheet for each category of tactic. For this worksheet, in column one, lists all the actions taken within one group of tactics. Then identify the five most significant factors, list their names in line 1. It is important to remember that factors are by definitions phenomena which no actor controls. Then ask whether this factor can affect the outcome of this particular action. Repeat this worksheet for each category of tactic which means that usually you will need to complete 4 or 5 of these.

Worksheet 19. Possible Key Factors	
Number	Possible Key Factor
1	

The Freedonian authorities would complete this worksheet as follows.

Worksheet 19. Possible Key Factors	
Number	Possible Key Factor
1	Natural disaster

WORKSHEET 20: KEY FACTORS BY TACTIC

This worksheet is completed as the previous worksheets have been.

Worksheet 20. Key Factors by Tactic	
Category of Tactic:	
Tactic	Can Key Factor 1 Affect? (Y/N)

For the Freedonian situation, the worksheet can be completed as follows.

Worksheet 20. Key Factors by Tactic	
Category of Tactic: crisis	
Tactic	Can Key Factor 1 Affect? (Y/N)
Realizes the shortages of certain supplies	Y
Realizes pandemic is creating several other major problems	Y

Worksheet 20. Key Factors by Tactic	
Category of Tactic: coping	
Tactic	Can Key Factor 1 Affect? (Y/N)
Works to respond to increased demand for certain supplies	Y
Delivers a financial health package to protect all Freedonians	Y
Expands subsidized telehealth services	Y
Supports Freedonians experiencing domestic, family, and sexual violence due to the fallout of coronavirus	Y
Funds mental health services	Y

Worksheet 20. Key Factors by Tactic	
Category of Tactic: planned	
Tactic	Can Key Factor 1 Affect? (Y/N)
Puts limits on some prescription and over the counter medications	Y

Worksheet 21: Tactical Goal

The next step is to identify the tactical goal to be attained. The last few worksheets require no instructions.

Worksheet 21. Tactical Goal					
Option	Description	Goal	Likelihood of success	Benefits	Costs
1					
2					

The Freedonian situation can be analyzed as follows.

Worksheet 21. Tactical Goal					
Option	Description	Goal	Likelihood of success	Benefits	Costs
1	Purchase	Get more supplies within a certain timeframe	50%	Greater certainty, even if there are shortages	Lost income Lost job creation
2	Manufacture	Get more supplies within a certain timeframe	40%	Local job creation Puts money into the local economy Once in place, assured supply long term	Delays costs lives Delays puts professionals more at risk

After that, the time has now come to design the next action to be taken in the crisis.

WORKSHEET 22: TACTIC DESIGN

Similarly, Worksheet 22 is self-explanatory.

The best moment to act is at a strategic node, where the success or failure of your strategy is at stake. It is possible to identify these nodes using Worksheet 7: Strategic Nodes. Once these nodes are identified, forecast each option you are considering, using Worksheet 23: Option by Node.

Worksheet 22. Tactic Design		
Tactical Goal:		
Option / Component	Option 1:	Option 2:
Time required		
Deadline		
Place		
Actor(s)		
Action		
Information needed		
Collaboration needed from		
Inaction needed from		
Other requirements		

The situation in Freedonia can be represented as follows

Worksheet 22. Tactic Design		
Tactical Goal:		
Option / Component	Option 1: buy	Option 2: manufacture
Time required	Delivery time from abroad	Setting up production and delivery chains
Deadline	3 months from order	3 months from order
Place	Seat of Freedonian government, location of foreign factories	Seat of Freedonian government, location of existing factories
Actor(s)	Foreign manufacturers	Freedonian manufacturers
Action	Negotiate purchase agreement, specifications, and delivery dates	Set up production and delivery chains to specifications
Information needed	Manufacturers, production volume, specifications of products, transportation time	Manufactures, production requirements, specifications of products, transportation time
Collaboration needed from	Manufacturers	Manufacturers
Inaction needed from	Other purchasers	Other purchasers
Other requirements	n/a	Sufficient domestic expertise Availability of components or materials

Worksheet 23: Options by Node

Once again, it is possible to cut and paste actions from an earlier worksheet.

Worksheet 23. Options by Node	
Strategic Node:	
Option 1:	Option 2:

For the purposes of illustration, we shall examine only the first crisis.

Worksheet 23. Options by Node	
Strategic Node: ____________realize shortages of certain supplies___	
Option 1: buy	Option 2: make
Find manufacturers	Find manufacturers
Learn production volume	Tender production work
Learn delivery times	Award contract
Place orders	Test prototypes for specifications
	Place order
	Wait for production
	Wait for delivery

Once this has been done, you can select the option or bundle of tactics you wish to adopt.

Worksheet 24: List of Individual Tactics

The next step is to list the tactics necessary within the category designated, with the Worksheet 24: List of Individual Tactics. In this case there will be a list of tactics for buying supplies.

Worksheet 24. List of Individual Tactics		
Number	Tactic	Description
1		
2		
3		
4		

In the Freedonian situation, we find as follows.

Worksheet 24. List of Individual Tactics		
Number	Tactic	Description
1	Find manufacturers	
2	Learn production volume	
3	Learn delivery times	
4	Place orders	

If the situation is simple enough to have only five tactics or less, you can skip the preceding and go directly to the next worksheet.

Worksheet 25: Design of Individual Tactics

At this point, it becomes possible to design each tactic within the category chosen, using Worksheet 25: Design of Individual Tactics.

Worksheet 25. Design of Individual Tactics.				
Tactic: _____buy supplies__________________				
Component	Tactic 1	Tactic 2	Tactic 3	Tactic 4
Action				
Actor				
Deadline				
Location				
Information needed				
Time needed				
Material needed				
Important Rules				

Worksheet 25. Design of Individual Tactics.				
Tactic: _____buy supplies_________________				
Component	Tactic 1	Tactic 2	Tactic 3	Tactic 4
Important People				

In the Freedonian situation, we find as follows.

Worksheet 25. Design of Individual Tactics.				
Tactic: buy supplies				
Component	Tactic 1	Tactic 2	Tactic 3	Tactic 4
Action	Find manufacturers	Learn production volume	Learn delivery times	Place orders
Actor	government	government	government	Government
Deadline				
Location	Seat of government	Seat of government	Seat of government	Seat of government
Information needed	Manufacturers of various equipment	Usual production volume of various equipment	Usual delivery times, back orders if any	Purchase protocols, internal and international
Time needed	1 week	1 week	1 week	1 week
Material needed	Office space and supplies, means of communication	Office space and supplies, means of communication	Office space and supplies, means of communication	Office space and supplies, means of communication
Important Rules	Financial accountability, contract law, collective agreements	Financial accountability, contract law, collective agreements	Financial accountability, contract law, collective agreements	Financial accountability, contract law, collective agreements
Important People	Public servants, manufacturers	Public servants, manufacturers	Public servants, manufacturers	Public servants, manufacturers

We can now move to the illustration of this method of analysis using a series of case studies moving from the individual to the group to the state and groups of states. Each case study includes a narrative of events, followed by the analysis using the worksheet method.

Chapter 4

Consumers of Health Services and Poverty

This semi-fictional case study takes the form of an activist's narrative.

How would the poor organize to get better health services? How could they? On an individual basis, individuals negotiate. Poor people may not be socialized to stand up for themselves and may therefore not be likely to do so. Indeed, the anti-poverty activists are for the most part middle class. Most poor people have no sense of their own power.

It took me years to come to understand what it meant to be poor, and even now I only have a dim understanding of it. To be mistreated, to be abused, to be battered, that I know about. But I'm from a privileged family. Poor was something other people were. Poor was my father who went to school without underwear because there was not enough money to buy it for all sixteen children. Poor was my father-in-law, who went hungry as a child. Poor was my grandmother, crying into the laundry when she learned she was pregnant for the seventh time, in 1932. Myself, I have never had not enough to eat. I do not remember ever going into a grocery store and not being able to buy anything I want. Most of all I don't remember ever thinking I was not entitled to have money. I was taught to strive, yes, and from an early age. No one ever told me I should be happy with a minimum-wage job.

So when I saw a musical about people on social assistance, put on as a fundraiser, I was shocked when a social worker said: "Yeah, that's what we would like the poor to be: happy, inventive, hardworking." The myth of social mobility was important to me. The first poor I met was a pregnant sixteen-year-old who wasn't sure who the father was in the days before DNA testing, living in social housing and learning she was pregnant when her breasts lactated and her mother said: "Ah, the cow's going to have a calf." To me, she was a creature from another planet. Those ten guys I met in a prison workshop, whose biggest problem was being poor and either drunk or high and doing something dumb and getting caught? They spoke a language I did not know.

There I was, with this how-to book in my hand, and good intentions in my heart. What was I going to do to help this bunch of poor immigrants in substandard housing and low-paying jobs convince the emergency ward to not dismiss the mothers when they came in with their sick children? Was I going to provide them with enough medication for a few days so that they had a chance to get to the pharmacy? Was I going to convince the powers that be that having to pay a minimum cost of $5 was too much for most of these people? Obviously not. They had asked me for help, and I had the tools on hand, but I was about to find out what they thought of it.

Luckily for me, the group had a natural leader, Seonida. She was on welfare as a single mother, and she knew what was what. She later registered in college and argued with the professor about her essays: she did not want to learn to write academese, she said, because she wanted to still be understood by ordinary people. I thought she was great. Seonida took me in hand.

"So, you have a book, and you took a course. So where do you think we should start?" "Well," I said, "we should get together a small team, five to seven people, and talk things over, and develop a strategy. We need to get people on that team who are familiar with each of the limiting factors we are likely to encounter." "So, what does that mean in English?" "We need people who know really well what obstacles we are likely to encounter. We need someone who knows how much money we can spend and how to spend it to get the biggest bang for the buck. We need someone who really understands the hospital decision-making system. That person would have previous experience or contacts. We need someone who can figure out how much this would cost the hospital and all the arguments that will come up against us. We need someone who understands the poor people and will be able to get them to work with us." "Well, that sure as hell won't be you," said Seonida. "The last thing we need is some big executive that has ten people working under them." I was wearing my suit from work, and a briefcase, and yes, my favorite heels with the little bows at the back. "When do we meet?" "Well, said Seonida, "How about next Thursday at 6, and we can all have pizza." Yeah, food, I thought. It's a great way to ensure attendance.

On Thursday, everyone straggled in for about an hour. I was distracted by that but Seonida was focused. Seonida had a strength of will and a comfort level telling other people what to do, someone who had the credibility to inspire the trust of the people. We met in what had once been the proud dining room of a Victorian house. Now, in this parvenu town, character homes were disdained in favor of newly built places. The group had gotten this place for a song – the plumbing did not work very well, but it didn't matter since no one lived here. Once in a while, the ancient pipes would burp, and a sewer smell, riper in the summer, would wrap itself around one of the meeting rooms… an appropriate sensory experience to go with the inevitable chaos of the proceedings. Everyone sat around on cushions, there being no one in the room over the age of 45. The arguing started almost immediately.

"Those frigging emergency room people, they ignore the ones that aren't dressed as well." I failed to say: who are you? They all knew each other, but I did not know anyone except Seonida. "No," said another, "they don't exactly ignore us, we just come in last on their list." "Well, what's the difference if you've got two other kids with you waiting, and they get hungry and tired or both…" "There's no point in telling them anything, they don't like us." "No, they don't," I said, "but they won't admit it. If we can find a way to get them a message, maybe they'll wise up." One of them acknowledged me. "Good idea, giving them a message. There's no point in preaching, so how about demonstrating?" Then they went right back to thinking out loud. "What are we going to do, give them an Academy Award for hypocrisy?" "The damn system was set up to look after everyone, but now they don't treat us the same way they treat each other."

Part of the problem was that they would not give poor folks the forms to fill out complaints about not being treated strictly in order of medical emergency. I mean, they all knew the difference between heart attacks and an ankle sprain. But within those categories, the nice, well-dressed people with highly responsible jobs were being treated first. If you were a waitress or a factory worker, tough. Unemployed? Tougher. God help you if the boss fired you for being late or absent one too many times…And when you finally got the attention of a nurse or a doctor, they were much more likely to dismiss the complaint with an aspirin and a "Call your own doctor." Well, the doctor shortage was so bad most poor people couldn't get a doctor, and there was only one clinic in a poor neighborhood that would only take the locals and even then, not if they had other doctors. Lately, the emergency managers had been approached because of this. But they had had said that they never had any complaints. Well, I guess not. The nurse with the complaint forms insisted on hearing about complaints herself, and only if she decided the 'complaint was founded,' would she hand out a form.

Seonida cut through the crap: "Are they going to listen to us if we embarrass them, or are they going to listen to us if we teach them something?" The chorus was instantaneous: "If we teach them." "What do you suggest, Seonida?" I said. "Should we invite them here to listen to us, and see what they have to say?" OK, so everyone laughed when I said that. "I'm not finished. We invite them to have their say, and they will give us the party line. But we convince them that we are now on their side, and simply would like to help them get their message out. So, they give us the forms and we hand them around to any place."

Good one, I thought. But the complaint person would smell rat, and she would never do it. That was the tricky part, and I said so. "Don't worry, we're not going to send you. The minute they meet you they'll smell a rat. You won't even be in the room, not to worry," said Seonida. That was a relief, I guess. "No, we'll have them over and we'll have Uchaz and Bill meet with them, both of them want to be RNA's, right?"

Uchaz and Bill. I had to wonder what Seonida was up to. They did not come across as quick-witted or fast on their feet. No, they seemed even a little goofy to me. However, I had already been put in my place three times in as many minutes. I wanted to retreat to the comfort of my office and the warmth of my illusions about myself. I would be right there with "I told you so" in about two weeks, when the whole thing fell apart.

I never did get to say those words. That was because our two yahoos, Uchaz and Bill had a gift, the gift of not seeming threatening. Now, I wouldn't know anything about that gift. I am a bulldozer. I am high-energy and I can't hide it. I wound up feeling envious, even a little jealous.

Uchaz and Bill went to meet with the complaint nurse. They said they were just trying to figure out the system. Uchaz said, truthfully, that she was about to go into nursing herself next September. The complaint nurse, who had the job because she had hurt herself in the workplace, was well disposed. Nurse Hodditt went through all the regulations that had to do with complaints. She explained the regulations to them, as well as the process involved, and talked about the role of the hospital as well as the College of Nurses and the College of Physicians. Uchaz and Bill did a particularly good job of really getting to understand the system, which was complicated. And then they asked for some pamphlets that explained the process of complaints, which they got. Two of them, one each. And then Uchaz and Bill left.

They were laughing when they told the group about it at the next meeting. Then they debated whether we should invite her, and people said they wanted to have her over. I couldn't imagine how we could meet with her and not reveal our plan. But I had underestimated everybody. I tossed twenty dollars at someone and told them to get what the locals called donut holes, the tiny round donuts made from the dough that was cut out of the middle of the donut. We would have something to pass around the table.

Nurse Hodditt came. Uchaz met her and shepherded her to our smelly little dining room. Uchaz had asked for and got us a presentation on the public and community relations office of the hospital. Nurse said she was glad to be there. I had drilled into everybody not to ask any pointed questions, just points of information, and they did that perfectly. She would not have any donuts, but she did have a cup of coffee. And as soon as we left, we went into a huddle.

The conclusions were obvious: there was no way we were going to change the regulations regarding treatment of complaints. There was no way we could make our point head on, it would be too easy for Nurse Hodditt to bypass us completely and not give out the forms. So, Bill said: "Let's ask her for some complaint sheets to explain to others in the community how it works, and 'what a great system it is'." Because our sharp-witted members had noticed that Nurse Hodditt had to record the number of inquiries and the number of complaints fielded. If the number of inquiries about the complaint system went up, but the number of actual complaints did not, because Hodditt didn't hand out any forms, she would still have to explain that. I didn't think it would work. I figured everyone would learn as much by failing as by succeeding. So, I said nothing. Good thing for me, because boy, was I wrong.

Bill and Uchaz went and met with Nurse Hodditt again, and said that as part of their little training they wanted to help make known the really good process in existence for complaints. To do that, they wanted to distribute some of the sheets as example and some of the pamphlets. Well, they got exactly five sheets with a big black line diagonally across the page, with 'Sample" in big black letters. But they got a case, a bushel of the pamphlets that they could distribute. And they did. They put them in food banks, homeless shelters, emergency rooms, community health clinics, welfare and unemployment offices, pawnbrokers, cheque-cashing places, the police station: everywhere where the least advantaged people congregate. Result: Nurse Hodditt was swamped with inquiries if not complaints, and her statistics were skewed for that quarter. I don't know how she rationalized it all to herself, but there was no escaping the conclusion: she was actively discouraging complaints. Even better, she had to report the inquiries by neighborhoods, in case there was evidence of ethnic bias. But the neighborhoods were all the poorer ones… Mission accomplished. And the group had achieved something that would have been impossible for me.

Worksheet 1. Strategy		
Issue/Problem	Poor people being treated differently in ER	
Goal	Make ER personnel aware of differential treatment using complaints	
Core idea (metaphor, slogan, etc.)	Praise to a point	
Tactics (actions or bundles of actions)	1	Praise nurse
	2	Obtain pamphlets
	3	Distribute pamphlets
	4	Make nurse aware of her limiting complaints

Worksheet 2. Key Actors	
All Actors	Can this actor affect your achieving the goal? (Yes or No)
Narrator	Y
Poor	Y
ER personnel	Y
Nurse Hodditt	Y
Anti-poverty activists	Y
Bill	Y
Uchaz	Y
Seonida	Y
Other patients in ER	N
10 men in prison	N
Pregnant sixteen-year-old	N
Children's Aid Society	N
Students	N
'powers that be' i.e., legislators	N
Hospital administrators	Y

Worksheet 3. An Actor's Actions and Tactics		
Actor: Bill		
Time/Date	Action	Is this a tactic? (Yes or No)
Not known	Says, along with everyone else: "If we teach them."	N
Not known	Laughs, along with everyone else.	N
Not known	Does not come across as quick-witted.	N
Not known	Does not come across as fast on his feet.	N
Not known	Seems a little goofy to narrator.	N
Not known	Has a gift of not seeming threatening.	Y
Not known	Goes to meet with the complaint nurse with Uchaz.	Y
Not known	Says to the nurse he and his buddy are just trying to figure out the system.	Y
Not known	Does a particularly good job of understanding the complaint system.	Y
Not known	Asks for some pamphlets.	Y
Not known	Leaves meeting with nurse Hodditt with Uchaz.	Y

Worksheet 3. An Actor's Actions and Tactics		
Actor: Bill		
Time/Date	Action	Is this a tactic? (Yes or No)
Not known	Laughs as he recounts meeting.	N
Not known	Participates in debate about inviting nurse Hodditt.	Y
Not known	Attends meeting in dining room with nurse Hodditt.	Y
Not known	Participates in huddle after meeting.	Y
Not known	Says: "let's ask her for some pamphlets."	Y
Not known	Noticed nurse Hodditt had to record number of inquiries as well as complaints.	Y
Not known	Meets with nurse Hodditt again with Uchaz.	Y
Not known	Says that they wanted to help make known the complaint process.	Y
Not known	Gets five sample complaint sheets.	Y
Not known	Gets a box of pamphlets.	Y
Not known	with Uchaz distributes pamphlets in food banks, homeless shelters, emergency rooms, community health clinics, welfare office, unemployment office, pawnbrokers, cheque-cashing businesses, police station.	Y

Worksheet 4. Resources a Strategy Can Draw On			
Resource	Do you have enough? (Y or N)	Is this a 'nice to have?'	Is this a 'must have'?
Narrator's book	Y	Y	
Narrator's knowledge	Y	Y	
Narrator's experience	Y	Y	
Team members other than Bill and Uchaz	Y		Y
Seonida's leadership	Y	Y	
Time to meet	Y		Y
Money for pizza	Y	Y	
Dining room of the Victorian house	Y		Y
Team members' experiences in ER	Y		Y
Seonida's facilitating skills	Y	Y	
Bill's gift of being unthreatening	Y	Y	
Bill's intelligence	Y		Y
Uchaz' intelligence	Y		Y
Bill's time to meet with nurse Hodditt	Y		Y
Uchaz' time to meet with nurse Hodditt	Y		Y
Nurse Hoddit's time	Y		Y
Nurse Hoddit's good will	N	Y	
Bill's time to distribute pamphlets	Y		Y
Uchaz's time to distribute pamphlets	Y		Y

Worksheet 5. What you can and cannot do		
Rule	Does this rule help you reach your goal?	Does breaking this rule guarantee your failure?
Rules about inquiries re: ER	Y	Y
Rules about complaints re: ER	N	N
Inquiries must be counted and reported	Y	Y
Complaints must be counted and reported	N	N
Courtesy	Y	N
Honesty	Y	N

Worksheet 6. Factors Outside Your Control			
Desired Strategic Outcome:			
Factors that help		Factors that do not help	
	→	←	COVID-19
	→	←	Natural disaster

Worksheet 7. Do or Die Moments		
Goal: Make ER Aware that they are discouraging complaints		
Steps to Goal	Problem 1	Problem 2
Seonida interacts with narrator ▼		
Seonida sees limitations of action led by narrator	Narrator lacks credibility with the poor ▼	
	Narrator withdraws from leadership role to advisor ▼	
	Seonida decides to call upon community of impoverished people	
		Participants start to argue almost immediately ▼
		Seonida harnesses information and will of participants ▼
Problem 3	Problem 4	Problem 5
Participants choose Bill and Uchaz to meet with Nurse Hodditt ▼		
Bill and Uchaz meet with Nurse Hodditt ▼		

Worksheet 7. Do or Die Moments		
	Nurse Hoddit controls access to complaint form ▼	
	Bill and Uchaz bring the information back to the participants ▼	
	Participants discuss the situation ▼	
	Bill realizes they could make their point by praising Nurse Hoddit	Bill and Uchaz praise the process in their second meeting with Nurse Hoddit ▼
		Bill and Uchaz receive many pamphlets from Nurse Hoddit ▼
		Bill and Uchaz distribute the pamphlets widely ▼
		The number of inquiries Nurse Hoddit receives increases significantly ▼

Use as many columns or rows as you need. When you are done:
BOLD or CIRCLE EACH DO-OR-DIE MOMENT.

Worksheet 8. Tactics and Counter Tactics			
Make ER personnel aware of differential treatment using complaints		Their Goal: Maintain complaint process to standards set by her superiors	
Your Tactics		Their Countervailing Tactics	
Says, along with everyone else: “If we teach them.”	→	←	Nurse Hoddit meets with Bill and Uchaz
Laughs, along with everyone else.	→	←	Nurse Hoddit controls access to complaint form
Does not come across as quick-witted	→	←	Nurse Hoddit keeps records of inquiries and complaints
Does not come across as fast on his feet.	→	←	Nurse Hoddit meets Bill, Uchaz a second time
Seems a little goofy to narrator	→	←	Nurse Hoddit receives Bill and Uchaz’s praise of the process
Has a gift of not seeming threatening	→	←	Nurse Hoddit gives Bill and Uchaz a box of pamphlets on the complaint process

Worksheet 8. Tactics and Counter Tactics			
Goes to meet with the complaint nurse with Uchaz	→	←	Nurse Hodditt receives a significantly increased number of inquiries
Says to the nurse he and his buddy are just trying to figure out the system	→	←	
Does a particularly good job of understanding the complaint system			
Asks for some pamphlets			
Leaves meeting with nurse Hodditt with Uchaz			
Laughs as he recounts meeting			
Participates in debate about inviting nurse Hodditt			
Attends meeting in dining room with nurse Hodditt			
Participates in huddle after meeting			
Says: "let's ask her for some pamphlets"			
Noticed nurse Hodditt had to record number of inquiries as well as complaints			
Meets with nurse Hodditt again with Uchaz			
Says that they wanted to help make known the complaint process			
Gets five sample complaint sheets			
Gets a box of pamphlets			
with Uchaz Distributes pamphlets in food banks, homeless shelters, emergency rooms, community health clinics, welfare office, unemployment office, pawnbrokers, cheque-cashing businesses, police station			

Worksheet 9. Core idea			
Category	Suggested Metaphors, Images, Analogies, Role Models	Your Metaphors, Images, etc.	Core idea
Military	Machine gun, rifle, tank	Target	Shoot down the complaint process with arrows of praise
Geographical	River, waterfall, creek		
Plant	Tree, fern, Venus flytrap		
Transportation	Bus, golf cart, car		

Worksheet 9. Core idea			
Category	Suggested Metaphors, Images, Analogies, Role Models	Your Metaphors, Images, etc.	Core idea
Sports	Caddy, gymnastics, football	judo	Use the complaint process's momentum to throw it to the floor
Mechanical	Wrench, Allen key, ratchet		
Insects	Mosquito, ant, butterfly	Mosquito	Prick the awareness of those handling complaints with inquiries
Animals	Cougar, puma, rhinoceros		
Role models	Princess Diana, Donald Trump, Gandhi		
Your own Category:	Your own metaphors:		

Worksheet 10. Nature of the Crisis	
Question	Answer (Y or N)
Do you have to change the values?	N
Choices are: Between self-orientation and community orientation? Between materialism and non-materialism?	 Community Non-materialism
Do you have to choose among the values for a priority?	N
Choices are: Self-orientations over materialism or non-materialism Community orientation over materialism or non-materialism Materialism over self-orientation or community orientation Non-materialism over self-orientation or community orientation	
Do you have to change the type of strategy?	Y
Choices are: To direct strategy of action To direct strategy of persuasion To indirect strategy of action To indirect strategy of persuasion	 X
Do you have to change the core idea?	N
Do you have to change the categories of tactics?	Y

Worksheet 11. Events Leading Up to Crisis				
Seonida interacts with narrator				
Seonida sees limitations of action led by narrator	Narrator lacks credibility with the poor			
	Narrator withdraws from leadership role to advisor			
	Seonida decides to call upon community of impoverished people			
		Participants start to argue almost immediately		
		Seonida harnesses information and will of participants		
		Participants choose Bill and Uchaz to meet with Nurse Hodditt		
		Bill and Uchaz meet with Nurse Hodditt		
			Bill and Uchaz realize Nurse Hodditt controls access to complaint form	
			Bill and Uchaz bring the information back to the participants	
			Participants discuss the situation	
			Bill realizes they could make their point by praising Nurse Hodditt	Bill and Uchaz praise the process in their second meeting with Nurse Hodditt
				Bill and Uchaz receive many

Worksheet 11. Events Leading Up to Crisis				
				pamphlets from Nurse Hodditt
				Bill and Uchaz distribute the pamphlets widely
				The number of inquiries Nurse Hodditt receives increases significantly

Worksheet 12. Tactics Before and During the Crisis		
Event	Type	Tactic
Seonida interacts with narrator	Planned	N
Seonida sees limitations of action led by narrator	Planned	N
Narrator lacks credibility with the poor	Planned	N
Narrator withdraws from leadership role to advisor	Planned	N
Seonida decides to call upon community of impoverished people	Planned	Y
Participants start to argue almost immediately	Planned	Y
Seonida harnesses information and will of participants	Planned	Y
Participants choose Bill and Uchaz to meet with Nurse Hodditt	Planned	Y
Bill and Uchaz meet with Nurse Hodditt	Planned	Y
Bill and Uchaz realize Nurse Hodditt controls access to complaint form	Crisis	Y
Bill and Uchaz bring the information back to the participants	Coping	Y
Participants discuss the situation	Coping	Y
Bill realizes they could make their point by praising Nurse Hodditt	Coping	Y
Bill and Uchaz praise the process in their second meeting with Nurse Hodditt	Coping	Y
Bill and Uchaz receive many pamphlets from Nurse Hodditt	Coping	Y
Bill and Uchaz distribute the pamphlets widely	Coping	Y
The number of inquiries Nurse Hodditt receives increases significantly	Outcome	N

Worksheet 13. Key Actors	
Number	Key Actors
1	Nurse Hodditt
2	Bill
3	Seonida
4	Uchaz
5	Participants in discussions

Worksheet 14. Key Actors by Tactic Category of Tactic: ____Planned__________________					
Tactic	Can Key Actor 1 Affect? (Y or N)	Can Key Actor 2 Affect? (Y or N)	Can Key Actor 3 Affect? (Y or N)	Can Key Actor 3 Affect? (Y or N)	Can Key Actor 3 Affect? (Y or N)
Seonida interacts with narrator	N	N	Y	N	N
Seonida sees limitations of action led by narrator	N	N	Y	N	N
Narrator lacks credibility with the poor	N	N	N	N	N
Narrator withdraws from leadership role to advisor	N	N	N	N	N
Seonida decides to call upon community of impoverished people	N	N	Y	N	N
Participants start to argue almost immediately	N	Y	Y	Y	Y
Seonida harnesses information and will of participants	N	Y	Y	Y	Y
Participants choose Bill and Uchaz to meet with Nurse Hodditt	N	Y	Y	Y	Y
Bill and Uchaz meet with Nurse Hodditt	Y	Y	N	Y	N

Worksheet 14. Key Actors by Tactic Category of Tactic: ____Crisis__________________					
Tactic	Can Key Actor 1 Affect? (Y or N)	Can Key Actor 2 Affect? (Y or N)	Can Key Actor 3 Affect? (Y or N)	Can Key Actor 3 Affect? (Y or N)	Can Key Actor 3 Affect? (Y or N)
Bill and Uchaz realize Nurse Hodditt controls access to complaint form	Y	N	N	N	N

Worksheet 14. Key Actors by Tactic Category of Tactic: ____Coping__________________					
Tactic	Can Key Actor 1 Affect? (Y or N)	Can Key Actor 2 Affect? (Y or N)	Can Key Actor 3 Affect? (Y or N)	Can Key Actor 3 Affect? (Y or N)	Can Key Actor 3 Affect? (Y or N)
Bill and Uchaz bring the information back to the participants	N	Y	Y	Y	N
Participants discuss the situation	N	Y	Y	Y	Y
Bill realizes they could make their point by praising Nurse Hodditt	N	Y	N	Y	N
Bill and Uchaz praise the process in their second meeting with Nurse Hodditt	Y	Y	N	Y	N
Bill and Uchaz receive many pamphlets from Nurse Hodditt	Y	Y	N	Y	N
Bill and Uchaz distribute the pamphlets widely	Y	Y	N	Y	N

Worksheet 15. Key Rules	
Number	Possible Key Rules
1	Rules about inquiries re: ER
2	Inquiries must be counted and reported

Worksheet 16. Key Rules by Tactic Category of Tactic: _____planned________		
Tactic	Can Key Rule 1 Affect? (Y or N)	Can Key Rule 2 Affect? (Y or N)
Seonida interacts with narrator	N	N
Seonida sees limitations of action led by narrator	N	N
Narrator lacks credibility with the poor	N	N
Narrator withdraws from leadership role to advisor	N	N
Seonida decides to call upon community of impoverished people	N	N
Participants start to argue almost immediately	Y	Y

Worksheet 16. Key Rules by Tactic Category of Tactic: _____planned________		
Seonida harnesses information and will of participants	N	N
Participants choose Bill and Uchaz to meet with Nurse Hodditt	N	N
Bill and Uchaz meet with Nurse Hodditt	Y	N

Worksheet 16. Key Rules by Tactic Category of Tactic: _____crisis________		
Tactic	Can Key Rule 1 Affect? (Y or N)	Can Key Rule 2 Affect? (Y or N)
Bill and Uchaz realize Nurse Hodditt controls access to complaint form	Y	Y

Worksheet 16. Key Rules by Tactic Category of Tactic: ____coping_________		
Tactic	Can Key Rule 1 Affect? (Y or N)	Can Key Rule 2 Affect? (Y or N)
Bill and Uchaz bring the information back to the participants	N	Y
Participants discuss the situation	Y	Y
Bill realizes they could make their point by praising Nurse Hodditt	N	N
Bill and Uchaz praise the process in their second meeting with Nurse Hodditt	N	N
Bill and Uchaz receive many pamphlets from Nurse Hodditt	Y	N
Bill and Uchaz distribute the pamphlets widely	N	N

Worksheet 17. Key Resources	
Number	Possible Key Resource
1	Team members other than Bill and Uchaz
2	Time to meet as a group
3	Team members' experiences in ER
4	Bill's and Uchaz's intelligence

Worksheet 17. Key Resources	
5	Bill and Uchaz' time to meet with nurse Hodditt

Worksheet 18. Key Resources by Tactic Category of Tactic: ____Planned___________________					
Tactic	Can Key Resource 1 Affect? (Y or N)	Can Key Resource 2 Affect? (Y or N)	Can Key Resource 3 Affect? (Y or N)	Can Key Resource 3 Affect? (Y or N)	Can Key Resource 3 Affect? (Y or N)
Seonida interacts with narrator	N	N	N	N	N
Seonida sees limitations of action led by narrator	N	N	N	N	N
Narrator lacks credibility with the poor	N	N	N	N	N
Narrator withdraws from leadership role to advisor	N	N	N	N	N
Seonida decides to call upon community of impoverished people	Y	Y	Y	N	Y
Participants start to argue almost immediately	Y	Y	Y	N	Y
Seonida harnesses information and will of participants	Y	Y	Y	Y	N
Participants choose Bill and Uchaz to meet with Nurse Hodditt	Y	Y	Y	Y	Y
Bill and Uchaz meet with Nurse Hodditt	N	N	N	Y	Y

Worksheet 18. Key Resources by Tactic Category of Tactic: ____Crisis___________________					
Tactic	Can Key Resource 1 Affect? (Y or N)	Can Key Resource 2 Affect? (Y or N)	Can Key Resource 3 Affect? (Y or N)	Can Key Resource 3 Affect? (Y or N)	Can Key Resource 3 Affect? (Y or N)
Bill and Uchaz realize Nurse Hodditt controls	N	N	N	Y	Y

Worksheet 18. Key Resources by Tactic Category of Tactic: ____Crisis____________________					
access to complaint form					

Worksheet 18. Key Resources by Tactic Category of Tactic: ____Coping____________________					
Tactic	Can Key Resource 1 Affect? (Y or N)	Can Key Resource 2 Affect? (Y or N)	Can Key Resource 3 Affect? (Y or N)	Can Key Resource 3 Affect? (Y or N)	Can Key Resource 3 Affect? (Y or N)
Bill and Uchaz bring the information back to the participants	Y	Y	Y	Y	Y
Participants discuss the situation	Y	Y	Y	N	Y
Bill realizes they could make their point by praising nurse Hodditt	Y	Y	Y	Y	N
Bill and Uchaz praise the process in their second meeting with Nurse Hodditt	N	N	N	Y	Y
Bill and Uchaz receive many pamphlets from Nurse Hodditt	N	N	N	Y	Y
Bill and Uchaz distribute the pamphlets widely	N	N	N	Y	Y

Worksheet 19. Possible Key Factors	
Number	Possible Key Factors
1	High mortality or morbidity contagious respiratory illness emerges
2	Natural disaster

Worksheet 20. Key Factors by Tactic Category of Tactic: planned		
Tactic	Can Key Factor 1 Affect? (Y or N)	Can Key Factor 2 Affect? (Y or N)
Seonida interacts with narrator	Y	Y

Worksheet 20. Key Factors by Tactic Category of Tactic: planned		
Seonida sees limitations of action led by narrator	N	Y
Narrator lacks credibility with the poor	N	Y
Narrator withdraws from leadership role to advisor	N	Y
Seonida decides to call upon community of impoverished people	Y	Y
Participants start to argue almost immediately	Y	Y
Seonida harnesses information and will of participants	N	Y
Participants choose Bill and Uchaz to meet with nurse Hodditt	N	Y
Bill and Uchaz meet with Nurse Hodditt	Y	Y

Worksheet 20. Key Factors by Tactic Category of Tactic: crisis		
Tactic	Can Key Factor 1 Affect? (Y or N)	Can Key Factor 2 Affect? (Y or N)
Bill and Uchaz realize Nurse Hodditt controls access to complaint form	N	N

Worksheet 20. Key Factors by Tactic Category of Tactic: coping		
Tactic	Can Key Factor 1 Affect? (Y or N)	Can Key Factor 2 Affect? (Y or N)
Bill and Uchaz bring the information back to the participants	Y	Y
Participants discuss the situation	Y	Y
Bill realizes they could make their point by praising Nurse Hodditt	N	Y
Bill and Uchaz praise the process in their second meeting with Nurse Hodditt	Y	Y
Bill and Uchaz receive many pamphlets from Nurse Hodditt	Y	Y
Bill and Uchaz distribute the pamphlets widely	Y	Y

Worksheet 21. Tactical Goal					
Option	Description	Goal	Likelihood of success	Benefits	Costs
1	Increase number of inquiries	Raise awareness of bias in process at	80%	Achieves part of the goal quickly and easily Low financial cost Takes less time	Takes less time May use up motivation of poor

Worksheet 21. Tactical Goal					
		inquiry stage			with only partial results
2	Increase number of complaints	Raise awareness of bias in process at complaint stage	10%	Achieves overall goal more quickly	Negatively affect belief of the poor in the system Takes more time Takes more organization May cost more financially

Worksheet 22. Tactic Design		
Component \ Option	Option 1: Increase number of inquiries	Option 2: Increase number of complaints
Time required	30 days	120 days
Deadline	n/a	n/a
Place	Dining room of Victorian house, nurse's office, location of food banks, homeless shelters, emergency rooms, community health clinics, welfare offices, unemployment offices, pawnbrokers, cheque-cashing paces, police station	Dining room of Victorian house, nurse's office, location of food banks, homeless shelters, emergency rooms, community health clinics, welfare offices, unemployment offices, pawnbrokers, cheque-cashing paces, police station
Actor(s)	Bill, Uchaz, Nurse Hodditt, narrator, Seonida, participants in discussion group	Bill, Uchaz, Nurse Hodditt, narrator, Seonida, participants in discussion group, poor members of community
Action	Distribute pamphlets, encourage inquiries from poor members of community	Distribute pamphlets, coach possible complainants on how to get forms, obtaining complaint forms, help complainants fill out form, hand in forms, follow up
Information needed	n/a	Specific instances of bad treatment of poor at emergency room
Collaboration needed from	Poor members of community	Poor members of community
Inaction needed from	n/a	n/a
Other requirements	n/a	n/a

Worksheet 23. Options by Node	
Node	Option
Bill and Uchaz realize Nurse Hodditt controls the number of complaints	Increase number of inquiries
	Increase number of complaints

Worksheet 24. List of Individual Tactics, Option 1		
Number	Tactic	Description
1	Distribute pamphlets	Make list of homeless shelters, food banks, community health clinics, emergency rooms, police stations Assign the right number of pamphlets per location Deliver pamphlets to each location
2	Encourage inquiries from poor members of community	Identify potential complainants Communicate with potential complainants about pamphlets and inquiries Coach potential complainants on how to make an inquiry Get commitment from potential complainants to inquire Follow up

Worksheet 24. List of Individual Tactics, Option 2		
Number	Tactic	Description
1	Distribute pamphlets	
2	Coach possible complainants on how to get form	
3	Obtain complaint forms	
4	Help complainants fill out forms	
5	Hand in forms	
6	Follow up	

Worksheet 25. Design of Individual Tactics Tactic: option 1		
Component	Tactic 1	Tactic 2
Action	Make list of homeless shelters, food banks, community health clinics, emergency rooms, police stations Assign the right number of pamphlets per location Deliver pamphlets to each location	Identify potential complainants Communicate with potential complainants about pamphlets and inquiries Coach potential complainants on how to make an inquiry Get commitment from potential complainants to inquire Follow up
Actor	Bill, Uchaz	Bill, Uchaz

Worksheet 25. Design of Individual Tactics Tactic: option 1		
Deadline	7 days	30 days
Location	various	Chosen for convenience of potential complainants; various
Information needed	n/a	Personal circumstances and experiences of potential complainants
Time needed	7 days	21 days
Material needed	Transportation to the various locations	Transportation to and from meetings with complainants, transportation to hand in form; computers or pens, envelopes, photocopies of form
Important Rules	No behavior that injures credibility	Rules governing inquiries
Important People	n/a	Complainants

Worksheet 25. Design of Individual Tactics Tactic: option 2						
Compo-nent	Tactic 1	Tactic 2	Tactic 3	Tactic 4	Tactic 5	Tactic 6
Action	Distribute pamphlets	Coach possible complainants on how to get form	Obtain complaint forms	Help complainants fill out forms	Hand in forms	Follow up
Actor	Bill Uchaz	Bill Uchaz Seonida	Possible complainants	Complainants Bill Uchaz Seonida	Compla-inants	Bill Uchaz
Deadline	30 days from start	50 days from start	60 days from start	70 days from start	80 days from start	120 days from start
Location	various	At complainants' convenience	Nurse's office	At complainants' convenience	Nurse's office	Dining room, Victorian House
Information needed	Location of various community organiza-tions	Thorough knowledge of form and information on inquiry and complaint process	Thorough knowledge of form and information on inquiry and complaint process	knowledge of form	Location of nurse's office, hours of operation	Contact information for compla-inants
Time needed	30 days	20 days	10 days	10 days	10 days	40 days

Worksheet 25. Design of Individual Tactics Tactic: option 2						
Material needed	Transportation	Computer, pens, paper and stationery, form, convenient location to meet	Phone or transportation to nurse's office	Computer, pens, paper and stationery, form, convenient location to meet	n/a	Technology to contact complainants
Important Rules	Hours of opening of various community locations	Treat complainants with respect Confidentiality	Respect conventions to protect credibility	Treat complainants with respect Confidentiality	Hours of operations, nurse's office or Emergency Room	Treat complainants with respect Confidentiality
Important People	n/a	complainants	Nurse Hodditt, complainants	complainants	Complainants	Nurse Hodditt

Chapter 5

AN INFRANATIONAL GROUP DEALS WITH OTHER INFRANATIONAL GROUPS

In this case study, we observe the interactions over time of the physicians' unions and the Freedonian government over delivery of health services.

The Freedonian health care system evolved into its present form over four and a half decades. Its initial implementation took place between 1947 and 1961, starting with hospital services being covered. It then progressed a decade later to include physician services as well. The insufficiencies of the system, however, were clear within a decade of its inception, and its first review was launched in 1980. Health care in Freedonia ranked among the best in the world, but the commission charged with the review warned that there were threats to the accessibility of care.

At the time that the insurance scheme was developed for Freedonia, the main services that needed to be insured were those of physicians and hospitals. The idea that technology would evolve so quickly that the costs and the possibilities would spiral out of sight had not yet occurred to anyone even remotely connected with health. The cohort of health and health-related services not covered by the system, such as dental care, physiotherapy, medication, psychological or social therapy, was large. Moreover, the physicians were at the apex of the entire system. Given these facts, it was no surprise that there was little flexibility in the system for increased outpatient services, for example, for which a hospital would not be paid in proportion to their cost. There were no provisions for long term or home care, and there were no provisions for ongoing changes to move to new and less expensive ways of delivering primary health care or primary health services. There was also no support for the increasingly complex medical decisions that needed to be made in the expanding world of professional services or technological possibilities, nor did training of professionals come to include preparation for the sorts of decisions the increasing medicalization of society brought. There was no time allocated for physicians to do more and more administration, which they resented, and for which they were not paid. Finally, there were insufficient provisions for sharing of information on patients, let alone moving towards health care that considered all that information.

Some of the characteristics of the Freedonian system were enshrined in law. One of these was that there be universal access of patients to health care. Another characteristic was that both physicians and hospitals be paid only from one source, i.e., from the public purse, not insurance schemes, nor the patients themselves. Private clinics and hospitals also survived, as did independent physicians. Most interesting of all was the payment mechanism, which, in the early days of health administration in Freedonia, was fee for service. It was the simplest and easiest way to start. There was not much forecasting in those early days, so that fee for service meant that each act performed for the patient was to be billed separately. It became clear that this method of funding created a perverse incentive to increase costs ever upward, even without the increase of population, changes in demographics, advances in diagnostic and treatment, or increases in environmentally fostered diseases. Similarly, there was every incentive for physicians to spend only the minimum time required for patients.

The solution envisaged at the time of crisis of health care rationing and funding occurred was to introduce certain conditions of work for physicians. These could have included a proportion of the time or the services provided, an issue which became acute after the COVID-19 pandemic. Another solution would have been to develop an alternative to paying physicians and hospitals per service performed. In the meantime, however, the physicians came to be seen both as the primary origin of all the costs of health care, and the rulers of it. In an early and crude attempt to limit the rising costs, the number of students enrolling in medical school was limited, so that the physicians were controlled in numbers. But the physicians were controlled neither in terms of their location or the types of services they provided. For the government, this method represented a tempting and eventually irresistible target for control and criticism. At the same time, the government sought to make physicians both scapegoats and gatekeepers. Meanwhile the unions representing doctors did a better job of protecting their income stream than their public image. Many noticed their affluence and they came to be resented for their power. All other health professionals, including nurses and nurse-practitioners, worked for a salary under defined conditions. The solution Freedonian administrators needed to propose was to take away the burden of administration, but the trick was to make the physicians feel only the care the government had for their greater satisfaction.

The first decade after the institution of the health insurance scheme saw many changes. The role of a nurse was changing from that of generalist to that of specialist. There was at that time an acute physician shortage: in cities, the ratio of population to physician was about 800 to one, and much worse in rural areas. The trend towards specialization meant there were even fewer physicians in primary care. The emphasis of the health sciences was overwhelmingly curative, with prevention and enhanced well-being never much more than marginal areas. In the 1970s, studies on reforming the health insurance scheme began. The first of these studies cited the expanded role of the nurse as a high priority for the health care system. The first projects in community-based care also came into being. The first nurse-practitioner program was established in neighboring Silenia a year after the institution of the health insurance scheme in Freedonia. Then, to cater to the populations living in the isolated mountain area of Freedonia, the first education program was developed.

In 1972, physicians' and nurses' associations issued a joint policy statement on the role of the nurse-practitioner, and later a second Freedonian Ministry of Health report recognized the role of the nurse in health promotion and disease prevention. Legislative changes necessary for the introduction of nurse-practitioners in primary care were proposed in 1975. By the close of the decade, however, the legislation needed to create paid positions for nurse-practitioners still did not exist. There was a noticeable lack of support from both medicine and nursing for the new practitioners. In 1983, the last of the training programs in Freedonian universities closed to admissions.

By the 1990s, it became glaringly obvious to all that there was a growing crisis in the health system. Having physicians at the power apex of the system had allowed for changes which in the end offered physicians the best conditions of work, rather than looking first to the needs of the population. This proved to be a powerful incentive to enter the ranks of the medical profession, whose numbers meanwhile were strictly regulated. However, once the generation of physicians who had known the pre-insurance days had passed from active practice, it became, and came to be perceived, as a more craven profession. The next generation of Freedonian physicians preferred shorter hours. They came to expect the favorable conditions of work that sprang from the under-regulation of medical practice. Eventually, doctors began to simply abandon the provision of services they found unpleasant, onerous, or simply cost-ineffective. Patients with complex or chronic conditions, the poor or homeless, people with multiple social problems, the elderly, and patients in long-term care were refused by physicians as their patients. More and more physicians chose not to have hospital privileges and worked only out of their offices. Hospitals came to be overwhelmed by both orphan patients and emergency room visits. Government and physicians were increasingly at odds. Physicians as a group wanted to make as much money as possible, and to keep as much freedom to practice as possible. The government's interest was to control costs and to provide service to the voting population. But the government was stymied by the physicians' power and its own fear of consequences at the ballot box if they took the physicians on.

Throughout this period, the Freedonian health system was neither flexible nor up to date and it was without mechanisms through which it could effectively deal with the multiple challenges it faced. Freedonians could not be turned away from emergency rooms, nor could they be prevented for the large proportion of 'well but worried' visits to the doctor. There was no system for triaging patients. There was no mechanism to limit or redistribute the health services, which were available in finite quantity. Patients never knew how much their care cost. And so, in these conditions of unlimited growth, health care came to be one of Freedonia's most important industries. For its part, the interests of the government were in getting reelected and in controlling costs. The Nursing Association, taking all of this into account, cannily proposed the re-introduction of the nurse-practitioner as the solution to the government's problems. The nurse-practitioner would be first and foremost a member of the primary care team in the provision of primary health care services.

In 1993, Rufus T. Firefly announced a new Nurse-Practitioner Initiative as part of improving access to primary health care. The project involved commissioning of major discussion papers including needs assessment and proposed roles. He then established a Steering Committee with five sub-committees: fiscal, publicity and public relations, placement and service patterns, laws and regulations, and education, to release its recommendations six months later. This committee supported the development of training programs of nurse-practitioners with funding for the first five years, as well as a five-year evaluation project. Within a year, a consortium of Freedonian universities had been created to develop a training program, with the first graduates coming within three years. The committee recommended legislative authority for nurse-practitioners, and the law was passed two years later. A year after that, the Ministry of Health released funds for twenty nurse-practitioners in community-based agencies, including community health centers and mountain nursing stations. From taking stock to delivering a thorough proposal to the government took the Association about fifteen years. In 1997, the nurse-practitioner designation was created, with the proclamation of the Expanded Nursing Services Act of Freedonia. Within four years of the proclamation, there were over 750 nurse-practitioners in Freedonia.

During this period, Freedonian physicians had developed a set of three unions, one representing the family physicians, one representing the medical residents, and one representing the specialists. Each had its own leadership and governance structure, and, by and large, their interests coincided enough that they would have achieved greater strength if they had banded together. As their position was being eroded, however, the unions failed to change either their tactics or their goals. The physician associations became tempted to please only their own constituencies, and the government cleverly gave them their head.

The head of the union of family physician, Gloria Teasdale, was a natural strategist. She quickly foresaw that the days of doctors dictating to the government were about to come to an end. Teasdale therefore threw her lot in with government, although also enduring several leadership challenges from within, and she cooperated with the government's efforts to renovate the health system. By doing so, she managed to secure several advantages for family physicians, and accumulated a significant amount of good will. The initiative of networking family physicians, most of whom had previously been sole practitioners, became known as the Teasdale program. The unions of residents and specialists, respectively, chose to fight the government's imposition of working conditions in court, a costly and time-consuming solution that catered to the more militant elements in the unions. Meanwhile, they had to live with changes about which they had opinions but no input.

The type of strategy adopted by Gloria Teasdale and the union of family physicians was dictated by the values held by the group. Family physicians in Freedonia preferred influence in the long term, over acquiring higher incomes in the short term. They put their own common good over the good of each individual physician. In other words, they were both communitarian and non-materialist, more interested in their quality of life than their profit margins. With these types of values, the union was likely to adopt an indirect strategy of persuasion, whose goal was to influence the outcome of government decisions by participating in the process, to a greater extent that the other two unions. Its tactics included cooperation with the government over the renovation of the health system, participation in prototype programs and cases; and embracing greater cooperation with non-physician health professionals. They hoped to reduce the hours worked without affecting their income levels, and to off load certain time-consuming tasks, such as administrative matters, to other salaried professionals. Their core idea was: "you don't attract flies with vinegar." Teasdale was also effective because most family physicians were pragmatic: not inclined to strategy themselves, they were focused on the advantages that could still be obtained.

The union of medical residents held more individualist and materialist values. Medical residents represented the most recent additions to the profession, and they reflected the change of attitude and organizational culture more than the other two physician groups. There were elements in the union who understood that the changes sought by the government could result in shorter work hours and a more sustainable lifestyle. But these people did not win out in the end. The union of medical residents, much like the specialists, adopted a direct strategy of action, whose goal was to prevent the government from changing their working conditions. They did not seem to realize the sensitivity of political decision-makers to the dissatisfaction of the population would remain until it became so widespread that there was political capital to be gained from taking them on. For once, politicians were both forward-looking and patient, that is exactly what came to pass. The tactics used by medical residents included legal action, and the use of the media to court public opinion, but both tactics failed. The medical specialists' strategy could pass for the residents. They were lulled by the mistaken thought that their expertise would grant them special powers.

The government's strategy, on the other hand was much broader in scope. Holding communitarian and non-materialistic values, it chose an indirect strategy of persuasion whose goal was to force the physicians into accepting conditions of work. It used many tactics. First, the government used a divide-and-conquer approach, taking full advantage of the split of physicians into three trade unions. It took care to negotiate separately with each of them. It also grand-fathered the changes in conditions of work as much as possible, so that the base of opposition even among physicians would be split between generations. The government carefully gauged public opinion. And the government also made sure it had the support of all the other regulated health professions in Freedonia, of which there were over thirty. The Freedonian Supreme Court had ruled that certain conditions of work imposed on the medical profession in the past were unfair restrictions of trade because the physicians were considered independent businesses under fee for service. Since it was clear that the physicians would inevitably resort to the courts, Firefly submitted his proposed laws for referrals to the highest court, ensuring they were proof against previous constitutional arguments.

The government was comprehensive in its approach. It broadened the scope of practice of other regulated health professions. It introduced measures to reduce pressure on the worst pressure points in the system: patients with complex continuing conditions, crowded emergency rooms, and waiting lists. Nurse-practitioners staffed emergency rooms, but also assisted physicians in their practice and carried their own patient loads in community health clinics. Being on salary, nurse-practitioners took the time to chart out complex conditions and carry out health care for patients in difficult circumstances. Since about half of the visits to family physicians were from worried but well patients, and the emergency rooms were very crowded, the government introduced its telehealth program in greater Freedonia, staffed with nurse-practitioners who could answer questions about whether visits to a physician or an emergency room were warranted. Available 24 hours a day, 365 days a year, it became such a great success that the staff had trouble keeping up with demand.

The Freedonian government used both the carrot and the stick in the crisis with physicians. This crisis started when the government had to legislate the doctors to work in regional emergency wards. Over time, despite generous financial incentives, the emergency rooms of Freedonia had had more and more trouble getting physicians to cover the shifts. The situation became so difficult that emergency rooms in regional hospitals were closed during part of the summer. The government tried to negotiate with the physicians, but to no avail. Then someone in the prime minister's own riding who was having a heart attack died in an ambulance, because the emergency room nearest him was closed, and he was being driven to another center forty-five minutes away. It suddenly became clear that Freedonians had had enough. The government announced that, the special law, modeled on a forty-year old anti-miner's strike measure. The government had been canny in crafting this law: it required the College of Physicians to establish a national list of physicians qualified to work in emergency rooms. All these physicians would be required to work a minimum number of shifts in emergency rooms so that all could stay open 24 hours a day. If a physician refused a shift, that physician would be fined $1000 each time, and would still be required to work the shift. If the unions of physicians defied the government's law, the heads of each union would be personally fined $5000 a day, while the unions themselves would be fined $25000 a day.

Emergency room schedules were filled within three days. Rufus T. Firefly then announced that the government was going to renovate the health system on the principle of the needs of the population rather than on the working conditions for physicians. While he personally hoped mediation would resolve the issues, the government certainly would not hesitate to extend the special law's mandate again. Gloria Teasdale's family practitioners cooperated with the government, and the other physicians accepted the new conditions of work even as they unsuccessfully challenged the laws in court.

Physicians naturally thought of leaving Freedonia for other, similar states, where there was no national health care system. To practice in another jurisdiction, however, physicians had to apply for a license, for which their administrative and professional files were reviewed. The government instituted a policy where physicians who had been trained at the expense of the state would have to repay those training expenses plus interest before leaving Freedonia. If physicians declined to make that repayment, then the government put an administrative notice on their files. This administrative notice stated only that there had been a problem with the administration of practice, although it did not suggest any problems with the practice of medicine. The result of this notice, however, was to preclude the physicians from easily obtaining a license to practice elsewhere.

The physicians were relieved to have the complex continuing cases or the multiple problem patients taken from them, along with a substantial administrative load, for which they were not paid and which they resented. Meanwhile, physicians were now required to offer health care seven days a week, 24 hours a day, with the additional support of nurse-practitioners, as well as being required to network with other physicians. Physicians were now salaried based on the number and type of patients in their practice. The government also created regional centers of expertise for various needs in health care, on an epidemiological basis.

Finally, the government removed some of the pressures on physicians making all administrative and ethical decisions by introducing a Freedonian National Health Council, charged with considering issues in health care. The council developed a plan in how to equalize the salaries and working conditions of all health professionals, doctors included, and how to expand the health care system for medication insurance and alternative care. The Association was careful to be well-represented there.

The analysis below examines the Freedonian government's strategy regarding physicians. It presents an additional interest, as the analysis will show, of two crises instead of one.

Worksheet 1. Strategy		
Issue/Problem	Physicians' pay and conditions of work	
Goal	Save money and improve availability of physician services	
Core idea (metaphor, slogan, etc.)	Do an end run around physicians	
Tactics (actions or bundles of actions)	1	Negotiate separately with the three physicians' unions
	2	Comprehensively substitute other services or practitioners for physician services
	3	Assess and use public opinion
	4	Take administrative measures necessary to limit physicians' resistance

Worksheet 2. Key Actors	
All Actors	Can this actor affect your achieving the goal? (Yes or No)
Freedonian government	Y
Physicians	Y
Hospitals	Y
1980 review commission	Y
Patients	Y
Medical students	Y
Other health professionals	Y
Nurses	Y
Nurse-practitioners	Y

Worksheet 2. Key Actors	
Physician unions	Y
Freedonian Professional Nursing Association	Y
Isolated Freedonian populations	Y
Patients with complex conditions	Y
Poor patients	Y
Patients with multiple social problems	Y
Elderly patients	Y
Minister of health, R.T. Firefly	Y
1993 Steering Committee	Y
Families of patients	Y
Union of family physicians	Y
Gloria Teasdale, head of union of family physicians	Y
Union of medical residents	Y
Freedonian Supreme Court	Y
Freedonian Prime minister	Y
College of Physicians	Y
Physicians qualified to work in Emergency Rooms	Y
Freedonian National Health Council	N

Worksheet 3. An Actor's Actions and Tactics		
Actor: Freedonian government		
Time/Date	Action	Is this a tactic? (Yes or No)
1947-61	Implements health system	N
	Enshrines some of the health system characteristics in law	N
	Establishes a fee-for-service payment system	N
	Fails to include large number of health and health-related services in coverage	N
1980	commissions review of health system	Y
	Does not support increasingly complex medical decision-making	N
	Does not have an effective information-sharing system	N
	Does not pay physicians for administrative work	N
	Sees physicians as the primary origin of all the costs of health care and the rulers of it	N
	Limits enrolment in medical schools	Y
	Has all health professionals but physicians work on salary under defined conditions	N
	Develops nurse-practitioner education program to cater to isolated populations	Y
	Recognizes influence of determinants of health	N
1983	Ends nurse-practitioner program because of over- supply of physicians	N

Worksheet 3. An Actor's Actions and Tactics		
	Is increasingly at odds with physicians over control of costs and provision of services to voters	N
	Allows conditions to exist where health care became of the country's most important industries	N
1993	Announces new nurse-practitioner initiative, major discussion papers, steering committee	Y
1997	Proclaims Expanded Nursing Services Act of Freedonia	Y
	Cooperates with Gloria Teasdale	Y
	Forces physicians into accepting conditions of work	Y
	Takes advantage of split of physicians into three unions	Y
	Negotiates separately with each union of physicians	Y
	Grandfathers change in conditions of work	Y
	Waits for public opinion to support its positions	Y
	Gets support of other health professionals	Y
	Consults with Supreme Court on constitutionality of proposed law	Y
	Used a comprehensive approach	Y
	Broadened scope of practice of other professions	Y
	Reduced pressure on system for complex conditions, crowded emergency rooms, waiting lists	Y
	Established telemedicine advice line	Y
	Used generous financial incentives to staff ER with physicians	Y
	Proposed a law to staff ERs	Y
	Announced it would use the same law to restructure the system using patient needs as a principle	Y
	Introduced Freedonian National Health Council to assist physicians in making administrative and ethical decisions	Y

Worksheet 4. Resources a Strategy Can Draw On			
Resource	Do you have enough? (Y or N)	Is this a 'nice to have?'	Is this a 'must have'?
Money to pay for health services and professionals	N		Y
Money to pay for training of health professionals	N		Y
Time to train health professionals	Y		Y
Time for physicians to work	Y		Y
Time to develop health care system 1947-1961	Y		Y
Time to review system 1980	Y	Y	
Information on health technology	Y	Y	
Information to support for increasingly complex medical decisions	Y		Y
Information on law and constitutionality	Y		Y

Worksheet 4. Resources a Strategy Can Draw On			
Information on methods of sharing patient information	Y	Y	
Information on forecasting	Y	Y	
Information on public perception of health care system	Y		Y
Information on public perception of physicians	Y		Y
Information on social determinants of health	Y	Y	
Information on health promotion	Y	Y	
Information on prevention	Y	Y	
Information on physician expectations	Y		Y
Information on demand for health care services	Y		Y
Information on services provided to patients	Y		Y
Strategic skills of union leaders	N	Y	
Strategic skills of government	Y		Y

Worksheet 5. What you can and cannot do		
Rule	Does this rule help you reach your goal?	Does breaking this rule guarantee your failure?
Freedonian Constitution	Y	Y
Scopes of practice for health professionals	Y	N
Expanded Nursing Services Act of Freedonia	Y	N
Special Law	Y	Y

Worksheet 6. Factors Outside Your Control			
Desired Strategic Outcome: save money and improve availability of physician services			
Factors that help		Factors that do not help	
	→	←	Natural disaster
	→	←	COVID-19 pandemic

Worksheet 7. Do or Die Moments		
Goal: save money and improve availability of physician services		
Steps to Goal	Problem 1	Problem 2
Is increasingly at odds with physicians over control of costs and provision of services to voters ▼		
Allows conditions to exist where health care became		

Worksheet 7. Do or Die Moments		
of the country's most important industries ▼		
Announces new nurse-practitioner initiative, major discussion papers, steering committee ▼		
Proclaims Expanded Nursing Services Act of Freedonia ▼		
Cooperates with Gloria Teasdale	Forces physicians into accepting conditions of work ▼	
	Takes advantage of split of physicians into three unions ▼	
	Negotiates separately with each union of physicians ▼	
	Grandfathers change in conditions of work ▼	
	Waits for public opinion to support its positions ▼	
	Gets support of other health professionals ▼	
	Consults with Supreme Court on constitutionality of proposed law ▼	
	Uses a comprehensive approach ▼	
	Broadens scope of practice of other professions ▼	
	Reduces pressure on system for complex conditions, crowded emergency rooms, waiting lists ▼	
	Establishes telemedicine advice line	Uses generous financial incentives to staff ER with physicians

Worksheet 7. Do or Die Moments		
		▼
		Proposes a law to staff ERs ▼
		Announces it would use the same law to restructure the system using patient needs as a principle ▼
		Introduces Freedonian National Health Council to assist physicians in making administrative and ethical decisions ▼

Use as many columns or rows as you need. When you are done:
BOLD or CIRCLE EACH DO-OR-DIE MOMENT.

Worksheet 8. Tactics and Counter Tactics			
Your Goal: save money and improve availability of physician services		Their Goal: protect the interests of family physicians	
Your Tactics		Their Countervailing Tactics	
Is increasingly at odds with physicians over control of costs and provision of services to voters	→	←	Cooperates with government
Allows conditions to exist where health care became of the country's most important industries	→	←	Negotiates separately from other two physician unions
Announces new nurse-practitioner initiative, major discussion papers, steering committee	→	←	
Proclaims Expanded Nursing Services Act of Freedonia	→	←	
Cooperates with Gloria Teasdale	→	←	
Forces physicians into accepting conditions of work	→	←	
Takes advantage of split of physicians into three unions	→	←	
Negotiates separately with each union of physicians	→	←	
Grandfathers change in conditions of work			
Waits for public opinion to support its positions			

Worksheet 8. Tactics and Counter Tactics			
Gets support of other health professionals			
Consults with Supreme Court on constitutionality of proposed law			
Used a comprehensive approach			
Broadened scope of practice of other professions			
Reduced pressure on system for complex conditions, crowded emergency rooms, waiting lists			
Established telemedicine advice line			
Used generous financial incentives to staff ER with physicians			
Proposed a law to staff ERs			
Announced it would use the same law to restructure the system using patient needs as a principle			
Introduced Freedonian National Health Council to assist physicians in making administrative and ethical decisions			

Worksheet 9. Core idea			
Category	Suggested Metaphors, Images, Analogies, Role Models	Your Metaphors, Images, etc.	Core idea
Military	Machine gun, rifle, tank		
Geographical	River, waterfall, creek		
Plant	Tree, fern, Venus flytrap		
Transportation	Bus, golf cart, car		
Sports	Caddy, gymnastics, football	vault	We will leap over the physicians
		football	We will do an end run around the physicians
Mechanical	Wrench, Allen key, ratchet		
Insects	Mosquito, ant, butterfly		
Animals	Cougar, puma, rhinoceros	kangaroo	We will jump over the physicians
Role models	Princess Diana, Donald Trump, Gandhi		
Your own Category: Building	Your own metaphors: dam, towers, bridges	dam	We will detour the river of physician services

Worksheet 10. Nature of the Crisis	
Question	Answer (Y or N)
Do you have to change the values?	N
Choices are: Between self-orientation and community orientation? Between materialism and non-materialism?	
Do you have to choose among the values for a priority?	N
Choices are: Self-orientations over materialism or non-materialism Community orientation over materialism or non-materialism Materialism over self-orientation or community orientation Non-materialism over self-orientation or community orientation	X
Do you have to change the type of strategy?	Y
Choices are: To direct strategy of action To direct strategy of persuasion To indirect strategy of action To indirect strategy of persuasion	X
Do you have to change the core idea?	Y
Do you have to change the categories of tactics?	Y

Worksheet 11. Events Leading Up to Crisis		
Event	Type	Tactic?
Implements health system		N
Enshrines some of the health system characteristics in law		N
Establishes a fee-for-service payment system		N
Fails to include large number of health and health-related services in coverage		N
Commissions review of health system	Planned	Y
Does not support increasingly complex medical decision-making		N
Does not have an effective information-sharing system		N
Does not pay physicians for administrative work		N
Sees physicians as the primary origin of all the costs of health care and the rulers of it		N
Limits enrolment in medical schools	Planned	Y
Has all health professionals but physicians work on salary under defined conditions	Planned	Y
Develops nurse-practitioner education program to cater to isolated populations	Planned	Y
Recognizes influence of determinants of health		N
Ends nurse-practitioner program because of over- supply of physicians	Planned	Y

Worksheet 12. Tactics Before and During the Crisis		
Event	Type	Tactic
Is increasingly at odds with physicians over control of costs and provision of services to voters	Crisis	N
Allows conditions to exist where health care became of the country's most important industries	Crisis	N
Announces new nurse-practitioner initiative, major discussion papers, steering committee	Coping	Y
Proclaims Expanded Nursing Services Act of Freedonia	Coping	Y
Cooperates with Gloria Teasdale	Coping	Y
Forces physicians into accepting conditions of work	Coping	Y
Takes advantage of split of physicians into three unions	Coping	Y
Negotiates separately with each union of physicians	Coping	Y
Grandfathers change in conditions of work	Coping	Y
Waits for public opinion to support its positions	Coping	Y
Gets support of other health professionals	Coping	Y
Consults with Supreme Court on constitutionality of proposed law	Coping	Y
Uses a comprehensive approach	Coping	Y
Broadens scope of practice of other professions	Coping	Y
Reduces pressure on system for complex conditions, crowded emergency rooms, waiting lists	Coping	Y
Establishes telemedicine advice line	Coping	Y
Uses generous financial incentives to staff ER with physicians	Crisis	Y
Proposes a law to staff ERs	Crisis	Y
Announces it would use the same law to restructure the system using patient needs as a principle	Crisis	Y
Introduces Freedonian National Health Council to assist physicians in making administrative and ethical decisions	Planned	Y

Worksheet 13. Key Actors	
Number	Key Actors
1	Freedonia government
2	Gloria Teasdale
3	Union of specialist physicians

Worksheet 14. Key Actors by Tactic
Category of Tactic: _________planned______________

Tactic	Can Key Actor 1 Affect? (Y or N)	Can Key Actor 2 Affect? (Y or N)	Can Key Actor 3 Affect? (Y or N)
Commissions review of health system	Y	N	N
Limits enrolment in medical schools	Y	Y	Y

Worksheet 14. Key Actors by Tactic Category of Tactic: _________planned_____________			
Has all health professionals but physicians work on salary under defined conditions	Y	N	N
Develops nurse-practitioner education program to cater to isolated populations	Y	N	N
Ends nurse-practitioner program because of over-supply of physicians	Y	Y	Y

Worksheet 14. Key Actors by Tactic Category of Tactic: _________crisis_____________			
Tactic	Can Key Actor 1 Affect? (Y or N)	Can Key Actor 2 Affect? (Y or N)	Can Key Actor 3 Affect? (Y or N)
Is increasingly at odds with physicians over control of costs and provision of services to voters	Y	Y	Y
Allows conditions to exist where health care became of the country's most important industries	Y	N	N
Uses generous financial incentives to staff ER with physicians	Y	N	Y
Proposes a law to staff ERs	Y	N	Y
Announces it would use the same law to restructure the system using patient needs as a principle	Y	Y	Y

Worksheet 14. Key Actors by Tactic Category of Tactic: _________coping_____________			
Tactic	Can Key Actor 1 Affect? (Y or N)	Can Key Actor 2 Affect? (Y or N)	Can Key Actor 3 Affect? (Y or N)
Announces new nurse-practitioner initiative, major discussion papers, steering committee	Y	Y	Y
Proclaims Expanded Nursing Services Act of Freedonia	Y	N	N
Cooperates with Gloria Teasdale	Y	Y	Y
Forces physicians into accepting conditions of work	Y	Y	Y
Takes advantage of split of physicians into three unions	Y	Y	Y
Negotiates separately with each union of physicians	Y	Y	Y
Grandfathers change in conditions of work	Y	Y	Y
Waits for public opinion to support its positions	Y	N	N
Gets support of other health professionals	Y	N	N
Consults with Supreme Court on constitutionality of proposed law	Y	N	N

Worksheet 14. Key Actors by Tactic Category of Tactic: ________coping_____________			
Uses a comprehensive approach	Y	N	N
Broadens scope of practice of other professions	Y	Y	Y
Reduces pressure on system for complex conditions, crowded emergency rooms, waiting lists	Y	Y	Y
Establishes telemedicine advice line	Y	Y	Y

Worksheet 15. Key Rules	
Number	Possible Key Rules
1	Freedonian Constitution
2	Scopes of practice for health professionals
3	Expanded Nursing Services Act of Freedonia
4	Special Law

Worksheet 16. Key Rules by Tactic Category of Tactic: _____planned________				
Tactic	Can Key Rule 1 Affect? (Y or N)	Can Key Rule 2 Affect? (Y or N)	Can Key Rule 3 Affect? (Y or N)	Can Key Rule 4 Affect? (Y or N)
Commissions review of health system	N	N	N	N
Limits enrolment in medical schools	N	N	N	N
Has all health professionals but physicians work on salary under defined conditions	Y	N	N	N
Develops nurse-practitioner education program to cater to isolated populations	N	Y	N	N
Ends nurse-practitioner program because of over- supply of physicians	N	N	N	N

Worksheet 16. Key Rules by Tactic Category of Tactic: ___crisis__________				
Tactic	Can Key Rule 1 Affect? (Y or N)	Can Key Rule 2 Affect? (Y or N)	Can Key Rule 3 Affect? (Y or N)	Can Key Rule 4 Affect? (Y or N)
Is increasingly at odds with physicians over control of costs	Y	Y	N	N

Worksheet 16. Key Rules by Tactic Category of Tactic: ___crisis__________				
and provision of services to voters				
Allows conditions to exist where health care became of the country's most important industries	N	N	N	N
Uses generous financial incentives to staff ER with physicians	Y	N	N	Y
Proposes a law to staff ERs	Y	N	N	Y
Announces it would use the same law to restructure the system using patient needs as a principle	Y	N	N	Y

Worksheet 16. Key Rules by Tactic Category of Tactic: _____coping________				
Tactic	Can Key Rule 1 Affect? (Y or N)	Can Key Rule 2 Affect? (Y or N)	Can Key Rule 3 Affect? (Y or N)	Can Key Rule 4 Affect? (Y or N)
Announces new nurse-practitioner initiative, major discussion papers, steering committee	N	Y	Y	Y
Proclaims Expanded Nursing Services Act of Freedonia	N	Y	Y	N
Cooperates with Gloria Teasdale	N	N	Y	Y
Forces physicians into accepting conditions of work	Y	N	Y	Y
Takes advantage of split of physicians into three unions	N	N	N	N
Negotiates separately with each union of physicians	N	N	N	Y
Grandfathers change in conditions of work	N	N	N	Y
Waits for public opinion to support its positions	N	N	Y	N
Gets support of other health professionals	N	Y	Y	Y
Consults with Supreme Court on constitutionality of proposed law	Y	N	N	Y
Uses a comprehensive approach	N	N	N	N
Broadens scope of practice of other professions	N	Y	Y	Y

Worksheet 16. Key Rules by Tactic Category of Tactic: _____coping________				
Reduces pressure on system for complex conditions, crowded emergency rooms, waiting lists	N	Y	Y	Y
Establishes telemedicine advice line	N	Y	Y	Y

Worksheet 17. Key Resources	
Number	Possible Key Resource
1	Money to pay for health services and professionals
2	Information on law and constitutionality
3	Strategic skills of union leaders
4	Strategic skills of government
5	Information on public opinion

Worksheet 18. Key Resources by Tactic Category of Tactic: _____planned_________					
Tactic	Can Key Resource 1 Affect? (Y or N)	Can Key Resource 2 Affect? (Y or N)	Can Key Resource 3 Affect? (Y or N)	Can Key Resource 4 Affect? (Y or N)	Can Key Resource 5 Affect? (Y or N)
Commissions review of health system	Y	N	Y	Y	Y
Limits enrolment in medical schools	Y	N	Y	Y	N
Has all health professionals but physicians work on salary under defined conditions	Y	N	Y	Y	N
Develops nurse-practitioner education program to cater to isolated populations	Y	N	N	Y	Y
Ends nurse-practitioner program because of over-supply of physicians	N	N	Y	Y	N

Worksheet 18. Key Resources by Tactic Category of Tactic: ____crisis___________					
Tactic	Can Key Resource 1	Can Key Resource 2	Can Key Resource 3	Can Key Resource 4	Can Key Resource 5

Worksheet 18. Key Resources by Tactic Category of Tactic: ____crisis__________					
	Affect? (Y or N)	Affect? (Y or N)	Affect? (Y or N)	Affect? (Y or N)	Affect? (Y or N)
Is increasingly at odds with physicians over control of costs and provision of services to voters	Y	N	Y	Y	N
Allows conditions to exist where health care became of the country's most important industries	Y	N	N	Y	Y
Uses generous financial incentives to staff ER with physicians	Y	N	Y	Y	N
Proposes a law to staff ERs	N	Y	Y	Y	Y
Announces it would use the same law to restructure the system using patient needs as a principle	N	Y	Y	Y	Y

Worksheet 18. Key Resources by Tactic Category of Tactic: _____coping_________					
Tactic	Can Key Resource 1 Affect? (Y or N)	Can Key Resource 2 Affect? (Y or N)	Can Key Resource 3 Affect? (Y or N)	Can Key Resource 4 Affect? (Y or N)	Can Key Resource 5 Affect? (Y or N)
Announces new nurse-practitioner initiative, major discussion papers, steering committee	Y	N	Y	Y	Y
Proclaims Expanded Nursing Services Act of Freedonia	N	Y	N	Y	Y

Worksheet 18. Key Resources by Tactic Category of Tactic: _____coping_________					
Cooperates with Gloria Teasdale	N	N	Y	Y	Y
Forces physicians into accepting conditions of work	Y	Y	Y	Y	Y
Takes advantage of split of physicians into three unions	Y	N	Y	Y	Y
Negotiates separately with each union of physicians	Y	N	Y	Y	Y
Grandfathers change in conditions of work	Y	N	Y	Y	Y
Waits for public opinion to support its positions	N	N	Y	Y	Y
Gets support of other health professionals	N	N	N	Y	N
Consults with Supreme Court on constitutionality of proposed law	N	Y	N	Y	N
Uses a comprehensive approach	Y	N	Y	Y	Y
Broadens scope of practice of other professions	Y	Y	N	Y	Y
Reduces pressure on system for complex conditions, crowded emergency rooms, waiting lists	Y	N	Y	Y	Y
Establishes telemedicine advice line	Y	N	Y	Y	Y

Worksheet 19. Possible Key Factors	
Number	Possible Key Factors
1	Natural disaster
2	COVID-19 pandemic

Worksheet 20. Key Factors by Tactic Category of Tactic: planned		
Tactic	Can Key Factor 1 Affect? (Y or N)	Can Key Factor 2 Affect? (Y or N)
Commissions review of health system	Y	Y
Limits enrolment in medical schools	N	Y
Has all health professionals but physicians work on salary under defined conditions	N	N
Develops nurse-practitioner education program to cater to isolated populations	Y	Y
Ends nurse-practitioner program because of over- supply of physicians	N	Y

Worksheet 20. Key Factors by Tactic Category of Tactic: crisis		
Tactic	Can Key Factor 1 Affect? (Y or N)	Can Key Factor 2 Affect? (Y or N)
Is increasingly at odds with physicians over control of costs and provision of services to voters	N	Y
Allows conditions to exist where health care became of the country's most important industries	N	Y
Uses generous financial incentives to staff ER with physicians	Y	Y
Proposes a law to staff ERs	Y	Y
Announces it would use the same law to restructure the system using patient needs as a principle	Y	Y

Worksheet 20. Key Factors by Tactic Category of Tactic: coping		
Tactic	Can Key Factor 1 Affect? (Y or N)	Can Key Factor 2 Affect? (Y or N)
Announces new nurse-practitioner initiative, major discussion papers, steering committee	Y	Y
Proclaims Expanded Nursing Services Act of Freedonia	Y	Y
Cooperates with Gloria Teasdale	N	Y
Forces physicians into accepting conditions of work	Y	Y
Takes advantage of split of physicians into three unions	N	N
Negotiates separately with each union of physicians	N	N

Worksheet 20. Key Factors by Tactic Category of Tactic: coping		
Grandfathers change in conditions of work	N	N
Waits for public opinion to support its positions	Y	Y
Gets support of other health professionals	Y	Y
Consults with Supreme Court on constitutionality of proposed law	N	N
Uses a comprehensive approach	N	Y
Broadens scope of practice of other professions	Y	Y
Reduces pressure on system for complex conditions, crowded emergency rooms, waiting lists	Y	Y
Establishes telemedicine advice line	Y	Y

Worksheet 21. Tactical Goal					
Option	Description	Goal	Likelihood of success	Benefits	Costs
1	Comprehensive approach	Bring about circumstances that will make physicians accept conditions of work	60%	Reserves use of special law for future use Keeps goodwill of physicians Fosters more team approach for increasingly complex health care	Takes time during which population fails to get services Higher pay for physicians, other professionals
2	Special law	Ensure provision of services to population by legislating conditions of work for physicians	100%	Quick Simple	Loses good will of physicians Addresses immediate problem but not increasing complexity of health care

Worksheet 22. Tactic Design		
Option / Component	Option 1:	Option 2:
Time required	12-18 months	3 months
Deadline	n/a	End of legislative session
Place	Freedonia	Freedonia
Actor(s)	Freedonia government, physician unions, unions of other professionals	Freedonia government, physician unions, Supreme Court of Freedonia

Worksheet 22. Tactic Design		
Action	Negotiate with health unions	Draft, refer, and pass special law
Information needed	Physicians' motivations and wants	Constitutionality of special law
Collaboration needed from	Unions in health care	n/a
Inaction needed from	n/a	n/a
Other requirements	n/a	n

Worksheet 23. Options by Node	
Options by Node	
Node	Option
Getting physicians to accept conditions of work	Comprehensive approach
	Special law
Staffing ERs with physicians	Special law

Worksheet 24. List of Individual Tactics, Option 1		
Number	Tactic	Description
1	Union cooperation	Cooperates with Gloria Teasdale
2	Exploits split	Takes advantage of split of physicians into three unions
3	Separate negotiations	Negotiates separately with each union of physicians
4	Grandfathering	Grandfathers change in conditions of work
5	Public support	Waits for public opinion to support its positions
6	Professionals' support	Gets support of other health professionals
7	Scope of practice	Broadens scope of practice of other professions
8	Easing bottlenecks	Reduces pressure on system for complex conditions, crowded emergency rooms, waiting lists
9	Telemedicine	Establishes telemedicine advice line

Worksheet 24. List of Individual Tactics, Option 2		
Number	Tactic	Description
1	Public support	Waits for public opinion to support its positions
2	Professionals' support	Gets support of other health professionals
3	Reference	Consults with Supreme Court on constitutionality of proposed law
4	Legislation preparation	Drafts law
5	Legislation adoption	Passes law

For the purposes of illustration, we will only analyze 5 of the actions. Public and professional support are analyzed for Option 2.

Worksheet 25. Design of Individual Tactics Tactic: option 1					
Component	Tactic 1	Tactic 2	Tactic 3	Tactic 4	Tactic 5
Action	Union cooperation	Exploits split	Grandfathering	Scope of practice	Easing bottlenecks
Actor	Govt of Freedonia	Govt of Freedonia	Govt of Freedonia	Govt of Freedonia	Govt of Freedonia
Deadline	n/a	n/a	n/a	n/a	n/a
Location	Freedonia	Freedonia	Freedonia	Freedonia	Freedonia
Information needed	Wants and aspirations of family physicians	Differing positions among physician unions	Previous grandfathering clauses	Existing scopes, possibilities of expanded scopes	Where the bottle necks are, what causes bottlenecks
Time needed	Several months	Several months	Several months	Several months	Several months
Material needed	Method of communication, meeting places	Method of communication, meeting places	Method of communication, meeting places	Method of communication, meeting places	Method of communication, meeting places
Important Rules	Previous and existing contracts, laws governing physicians' work	Previous and existing contracts, laws governing physicians' work	Laws affecting grandfathering	Laws governing scopes of practice of all health professions	Laws, policies, regulations in health care delivery
Important People	Union membership, public, Gloria Teasdale	Union leadership	Union leadership	Other health professionals' unions	Health professionals

Worksheet 25. Design of Individual Tactics Tactic: option 2					
Component	Tactic 1	Tactic 2	Tactic 3	Tactic 4	Tactic 5
Action	Public support	Professionals' support	Reference	Legislation preparation	Legislation adoption
Actor	Govt of Freedonia	Govt of Freedonia	Govt of Freedonia	Govt of Freedonia	Govt of Freedonia
Deadline	n/a	n/a	n/a	n/a	n/a
Location	Freedonia	Freedonia	Freedonia	Freedonia	Freedonia
Information needed	Results of public opinion polls	Positions of various professional unions	Constitutionality of law; requirements for a reference; Supreme Court calendar	Freedonian legal framework	Timetable and procedures for legislature to adopt laws

Worksheet 25. Design of Individual Tactics Tactic: option 2					
Time needed	1 month	3 months	6 months	6 months	3 months
Material needed	Office space and supplies, methods of communication	Office space and supplies, methods of communication	Office space and supplies, methods of communication, meeting place for justices	Office space and supplies, methods of communication	Office space and supplies, methods of communication, legislature meeting place
Important Rules	Regulations, laws, policies governing public opinion polls	Union constitutions	Constitution of Freedonia, procedures of Supreme Court	Laws of Freedonia	Legislative procedures
Important People	pollsters	Union leadership	Justices	Government lawyers	Legislators

Chapter 6

An Infranational Group Deals with a Supranational Group

A humanitarian, health-related national society deals with the international federation of similar societies, when the national government orders it to abandon part of its mandate after a scandal: this case study presents the problem without the solution adopted by the key actors.

The Freedonian Blue Cloud is that very volunteer-based humanitarian organization. The first Blue Cloud society was created after Luigi San Giacomo had a religious vision in 1874. Following the founder's vision, the Blue Cloud has worked to help people in times of peace to strengthen their capacities to live healthier lives and avoid conflicts and disasters. It grew to a global movement coordinated through the International Network, based in Gubbio, Italy, after a commission was set up in 1919 by a consortium of humanitarian societies to study how San Giacomo's vision might be implemented. The five members of the commission went on to become the founders of the International Network, inviting twenty states to participate in a conference to establish it. Today, the International Network enters conflict or disaster areas and negotiates on behalf of the wounded, combatants, and civilians in need of relief.

Freedonia's Blue Cloud was founded in 1904 by a military physician active in a unit putting down a rebellion in Freedonia's isolated mountainous regions. In 1909, the Freedonian government passed the Freedonian Blue Cloud Act, and shortly thereafter the flag of the Blue Cloud flew above a horse-drawn wagon used to transport the sick safely through a battle in the civil war. Freedonia, meanwhile, had already begun a program of health education to the public unlinked to either war or disaster. In 1947, the Freedonian Blue Cloud was charged with the national immunization programs. The Blue Cloud continues to provide this service for several decades.

At this time, the Freedonian Blue Cloud had 22 regions and 370 branches, including 7 000 staff and over 70 000 volunteers. The annual revenues before the close of the vaccination services was $200 million (US). In 2002, the Freedonian Blue Cloud provided disaster relief and humanitarian service to the public through its international, disaster, safety and community-based health and social services. It provided over $20 million (US) in international relief operations and over $10 million (US) in international development assistance. It trained nearly 50 000 people in disaster services, over 10% of the population in first aid, and 7 000 in emergency preparedness programs. Its vaccination initiatives include the creation of 50 branch offices, including over 5 million people vaccinated.

The Freedonian Blue Cloud became part of the International Network early, guided by the principles of humanity, impartiality, neutrality, independence, volunteerism, unity, and universality. It took great pride in serving anyone's needs, regardless of race, political beliefs, religion, social status, or culture. The goal of the Freedonian Blue Cloud always was to assist people deal with situations that threaten their survival and safety, their security and well-being, and their human dignity in Freedonia and elsewhere, as requested by the International Network.

The International Network

The International Network's slogan is "In fairness to all." The network makes no distinction among various nationalities, races, religious beliefs, socio-economic classes, or political opinions. It seeks to relieve the suffering of individuals, being guided solely by their needs, and to give priority to the most urgent cases of distress. The International Network was founded, as we have seen, in 1919 in Paris in the aftermath of World War I. The war had shown a need for close cooperation between societies, which, through their humanitarian activities on behalf of victims of war and disaster, had attracted millions of volunteers and built a large body of expertise. The first objective of the network was to improve the health of people in countries that had suffered greatly during the four years of the war. The network's programs came to rest in into four main areas: promoting humanitarian principles and values; disaster response; disaster preparedness; and health and care in the community. Health promotion came to represent the largest portion of the work, with assistance to around 30 million people annually since 1974. Health and community care have in recent decades become a cornerstone of humanitarian assistance, and now account for a large part of the network's spending.

The network is strictly neutral. It does not take sides in hostilities or engage in controversies of a political, racial, religious, or ideological nature. The national societies must always maintain their autonomy, to preserve their freedom of action so that they may be able to act in accordance with the principles of the network. The network made public its twenty-year strategy in 2000. It also defines three directions for the network and its member societies. First, member society programs should respond to local vulnerability and should focus on the areas where they can add greatest value. Second, the core areas of endeavor are the promotion of humanitarian values and principles, disaster response, disaster preparedness, and health and care in the community. Third, member societies should mobilize support and carry out their humanitarian mission while contributing to the building of civil society.

Cooperation between societies gives the network greater potential to develop capacities and assist those most in need. The role of the secretariat is to coordinate and mobilize relief assistance for international emergencies, promote cooperation between societies and represent them in the international field. The role of the field delegations is, first, to assist and advise societies with relief operations and development programs, and second, to encourage regional cooperation.

The network also leads one of the premier vaccination services in the world today. The reasons for such a priority are obvious: infectious diseases kill 13 million people every year. The combined effects of HIV/AIDS, tuberculosis, malaria, and water and sanitation-related diseases cause more deaths and destroy more livelihoods than natural disasters and conflicts together. Poverty is the primary cause of the spread of these diseases. The lack of information and access to services for the three billion people living on less than $2 (US) per day means they suffer the most. It is the role of the government to ensure that its health and social welfare system meets the needs of its population, particularly the most vulnerable.

Relations between the network and the member societies are governed by rules. Policies provide detailed direction for the network's humanitarian action in specific areas. They serve as a point of reference to ensure consistency in decision-making worldwide. The various policies define the boundaries for the conduct of the network and the people working within it. A permanent policy review process is always streamlining and revising existing policies to enable both the network and its member Societies to communicate the same messages worldwide. All member Society and network staff, delegates, and volunteers must be able to access, understand, and implement these policies. The authorities, agencies, and organizations with whom the member Societies and the network cooperate must be aware of the nature and content of these policies. The network increasingly involves member Societies in establishing and reviewing policies: that ensures that policies are appropriate. The network also holds that this gives member Societies ownership of these policies and a will to implement them. In addition, member Societies can use network policies as a basis to develop their own, more detailed policies which can then consider local needs, constraints, and relationships.

Network policy areas include:

- Programs and services: essential drugs and medical supplies, and first aid.
- Health: vaccinations, HIV/AIDS.
- Social welfare and youth.
- Emergency response: disaster preparedness, emergency response, food aid and nutrition, and post-emergency rehabilitation.
- Institutional capacity: development cooperation, development.
- Human resources: gender, volunteering policy.

In addition, the network operates according to its Constitution and rules of procedures. The network's Constitution includes the fundamental principles and general provisions such as the object and functions of the network, It includes articles governing membership in the network, such as duties and admission; regulations about the collective bodies of the network like the General Assembly and the secretariat; articles governing the actions of individuals in preeminent positions for the network, like the president and secretary-general; and three additional sections on elections, finances, and cooperation. The rules of procedures include rules on admission and suspension of members, the General Assembly, elections, the governing board and secretary general, the finance commission, regional conferences, and financial regulations.

Then disaster struck Freedonia's Blue Cloud. Between 1984 and 1992, several people were infected with rare diseases through improperly prepared vaccines, which carried newly mutated viruses. As tests to detect the new viruses were perfected, the vaccine supply became safe again, but people had died. The Freedonian government was forced to develop a compensation package for the sufferers. In 1993, the Blue Cloud welcomed the announcement of a public inquiry into Freedonia's vaccination system. The inquiry reviewed on the mandate, organization, management, operations, financing, and regulation of all elements of the Freedonian vaccine system, including the contamination of the supply in the mid-1980s and early 1990s. Corruption had played a part. The society cooperated fully in this process, seeing it as an opportunity for clarifying its role and responsibilities of the participants in the system. In 1997, the vaccine system was turned over to the newly created Freedonian Vaccine Services Association. This, in turn, created a problem of unity for the International Network, which now had to deal with two societies on the same national territory.

After the vaccine scandal, however, it was anxious to obey the government laws and move forward with the balance of its mandate, improving the health of vulnerable people through three strategic pillars:

1. Advocacy: through mobilizing people and influencing decision-makers - whether through private face-to-face advocacy or public campaigns - and through delivering services. It emphasized HIV/AIDS and on the role of volunteers in first aid, psychological support, and, more generally, in mobilizing the community to achieve greater equality of health outcomes.
2. Building capacity to bridge gaps: since there is always a gap between vulnerable individuals and households and the formal health and social welfare system, it operates through a network of volunteers that work inside vulnerable communities, putting knowledge and tools in the hands of the people, reducing vulnerability in the population and building caring communities.
3. Broadening interventions in crises: when the formal health system collapses due to a natural disaster, the Freedonian Blue Cloud assumes, on a temporary basis, a more comprehensive approach to health care than they do in non-crisis periods. While doing so, it supports coverage by the formal systems of health activities that go beyond those highlighted above, and for which the Blue Cloud has a comparative advantage.
4. Participating in an International Network's collective strategy: in doing so, Blue Cloud builds on lessons learned other regions; provides support for country plans with special consideration provided to scaling up programs to prevent/control communicable

diseases in a way that builds overall health capacity; and builds partnerships with national and international institutions to address global health issues.

5. Quality assurance in service delivery: to ensure that the Freedonian Blue Cloud services and training continue to save lives and minimize the effects of accidents or ill health, it will strengthen its collaboration with academic and medical institutions to standardize and improve life-saving techniques, tools and first aid products with research-based evidence.

One of the basic principles of the network is that there can only be one Blue Cloud or Blue Star society in any one country. That society must be open to all, and it must carry on its humanitarian work throughout its territory. The network is worldwide, and all member Societies have equal status and share equal responsibilities and duties in helping each other. However, the network, through its interim plan "Strategy 2010" has identified two goals that build on their comparative advantages and capacity to complement other national and local efforts. But Freedonia now has two societies, not one.

The network thinks of the national organizations as partners. The network uses these partners to strengthen the capacities of societies worldwide and ensure that this assistance is sustainable and consistent. At a local and regional level, member societies build partnerships with community groups, businesses, government ministries, and inter-governmental agencies, to enable them to integrate their programs and services in each country more effectively. Guiding and supporting the development of its member societies is one of the network's fundamental actions. It also creates the opportunity for member societies to work together. It also influences the behavior of those working within the Blue Cloud societies, public and private authorities, and members of the communities where Blue Cloud works to promote humanitarianism.

Given the unity of values, goals and tactics between them, the type of interaction between the network and the member Society, therefore, should be synergistic.

Worksheet 1. Strategy		
Issue/Problem	Freedonian Blue Cloud being divided into two societies	
Goal	Continue to work with International Network	
Core idea (metaphor, slogan, etc.)	In fairness to all	
Tactics (actions or bundles of actions)	1	Work will all International Network principles
	2	Respect for network policies and procedures for partnership
	3	Respect for domestic laws

Worksheet 2. Key Actors	
All Actors	Can this actor affect your achieving the goal? (Yes or No)
The Freedonian Blue Cloud	Y
Freedonian public	N
Freedonian disaster-trained people	Y
Blue cloud Vaccination Branch offices	Y
Freedonian Vaccinated people	N
Blue Cloud regions	Y
Blue Cloud staff	Y
Blue cloud volunteers	Y
Blue Cloud International Network	Y
First Blue Cloud society in history	N
Luigi san Giacomo	N
Other humanitarian societies	Y
Freedonian Blue Cloud founder	N
Wounded in conflict zones	N
Civilians in conflict zones	N
Combatants in conflict zones	N
Civilians in disaster zones	N
Founding members of International Network	N
Freedonian Government	Y
Rebels in Freedonia's mountain region	N
Freedonian hospital associations	Y
Freedonian provincial departments of health	Y
Freedonians infected in improperly prepared vaccines	N
Freedonians killed by improperly prepared vaccines	N
Freedonian inquiry commission into Blue Cloud vaccinations	N
Freedonian Vaccine Services Association	Y
Freedonian government decision-makers	Y
Freedonian health care system	Y
Freedonian national institutions	Y
International institutions	Y
Freedonian academic institutions	Y

Worksheet 2. Key Actors	
Freedonian medical institutions	Y
International Network member societies	Y
Secretariat of International Network	Y
Field delegations of International Network	Y
Government ministries of recipient countries	Y
Community groups of recipient countries	Y
Businesses of recipient countries	Y

Of interest here is that the case study does not list the International Network's actions in chronological order. Many of the actions have unknown dates.

Worksheet 3. An Actor's Actions and Tactics		
Actor: Freedonian Blue Cloud		
Time/Date	Action	Is this a tactic? (Yes or No)
1904	Comes into being, founded by a military physician	N
	Acquires legal status through Freedonian Blue Cloud Act	N
	Joins International Network early	Y
	Adopts International Network's principles of neutrality	Y
1920s	Organizes global health improvement program	N
1947	Begins national immunization programs in 1947	N
	Provides immunization for four decades	N
1984-92	Sickens and kill some people with its improperly prepared vaccines	N
	Welcomes a government inquiry	Y
	Accepts loss of its vaccination programs to the newly created Freedonian vaccine services Association	Y
	Moves forward with its remaining objectives in humanitarianism	Y
	Formulates three strategic pillars of advocacy, capacity building, and crisis intervention	Y

Worksheet 4. Resources a Strategy Can Draw On			
Resource	Do you have enough? (Y or N)	Is this a 'nice to have?'	Is this a 'must have'?
Information on controversies in recipient states	Y	N	N
Information on conflicts in recipient states	Y	N	N

Worksheet 4. Resources a Strategy Can Draw On			
Information on race in recipient states	Y	N	N
Information on political beliefs in recipient states	Y	N	N
Information on religion in recipient states	Y	N	N
Information on social status in recipient states	Y	N	N
Information on culture in recipient states	Y	N	N
Information on laws in recipient states	Y	N	Y
Information on health in recipient states	Y	N	Y
Information on most urgent cases of distress	N	N	N
Volunteers	N	N	Y
Expertise developed through operations	Y	Y	N
Money for staff	N	N	Y
Money for coordination	N	N	Y
Money for supplies	N	N	Y
Money for transportation	N	N	Y
Money for volunteer expenses	N	N	Y
Autonomy of national societies	Y	N	Y
Information on views of member societies	Y	Y	N
Information on trends in external environment	Y	Y	N

Worksheet 5. What you can and cannot do		
Rule	Does this rule help you reach your goal?	Does breaking this rule guarantee your failure?
Laws of national society states	Y	Y
International treaties relevant to conflicts	Y	Y
Laws of recipient states	Y	Y
Policies of national society states	Y	N
Policies of International Network	Y	N
Constitution of International Network	Y	N
Procedures of International Network	Y	N
International treaties relevant to disaster relief	Y	Y

Worksheet 6. Factors Outside Your Control			
Desired Strategic Outcome: continuing to work with in Freedonia			
Factors that help		Factors that do not help	
	→	←	Natural disaster
	→	←	COVID-19 pandemic

Worksheet 7. Do or Die Moments	
Goal: continuing to work in Freedonia	
Steps to Goal	Problem 1
Comes into being, founded by a military physician ▼	
Acquires legal status through Freedonian Blue Cloud Act ▼	
Joins International Network early ▼	
Adopts International Network's principles of neutrality ▼	
Organizes global health improvement program ▼	
Begins national immunization programs in 1947 ▼	
Provides immunization for four decades ▼	
	Sickens and kill some people with its improperly prepared vaccines ▼
	Welcomes a government inquiry ▼
	Accepts loss of its vaccination programs to the newly created Freedonian vaccine services Association ▼
	Moves forward with its remaining objectives in humanitarianism ▼
	Formulates three strategic pillars of advocacy, capacity building, and crisis intervention ▼

Use as many columns or rows as you need. When you are done:
BOLD or CIRCLE EACH DO-OR-DIE MOMENT.

Worksheet 8. Tactics and Counter Tactics			
Your Goal: remain part of International Network		Their Goal: Continue to work in Freedonia	
Your Tactics		Their Countervailing Tactics	
Comes into being, founded by a military physician	→	←	Invites 20 states to establish network
Acquires legal status through Freedonian Blue Cloud Act	→	←	Coordinates global Blue Cloud movement
Joins International Network early	→	←	Enters conflict zones and disaster areas
Adopts International Network's principles of neutrality	→	←	Negotiates on behalf of wounded, combatants, civilians
Organizes global health improvement program	→	←	Uses principles of humanity, impartiality, neutrality, independence, volunteerism, unity, and universality
Begins national immunization programs in 1947	→	←	Takes pride in serving anyone's needs, regardless of race, political beliefs, religion, social status, or culture
Provides immunization for four decades	→	←	Makes no distinction among various nationalities, races, religious beliefs, socio-economic classes, or political opinions
Sickens and kill some people with its improperly prepared vaccines	→	←	Seeks to relieve the suffering of individuals, being guided solely by their needs, and to give priority to the most urgent cases of distress
Welcomes a government inquiry	→	←	Sets first objective of the network as improving health of people in countries that had suffered greatly during the four years of the war
Accepts loss of its vaccination programs to the newly created Freedonian vaccine services Association	→	←	Developed programs in promoting humanitarian principles and values; disaster response; disaster preparedness; and health and care in the community
Moves forward with its remaining objectives in humanitarianism	→	←	Assists 30 million people annually in health promotion
Formulates three strategic pillars of advocacy, capacity building, and crisis intervention	→	←	Is strictly neutral
	→	←	Enables communities to reduce their vulnerability to disease
	→	←	Enables communities to prepare for and respond to public health crises
	→	←	Does not take sides in hostilities

Worksheet 8. Tactics and Counter Tactics			
	→	←	Does not engage in controversies of a political, racial, religious, or ideological nature
	→	←	Maintains the autonomy of all national societies
	→	←	Allows only one society per country
	→	←	Works worldwide
	→	←	Requires national societies to work on their entire territory
	→	←	Requires national societies to be open to all
	→	←	Faces problem of unity when Freedonian Blue Cloud cedes vaccination functions to new society
	→	←	Requires national societies to respond to local vulnerability
	→	←	Requires national societies to focus on areas where they add greatest value
	→	←	Defines four core areas of endeavor
	→	←	Requires member societies to contribute to the building of civil society
	→	←	Uses cooperation of national societies to develop capacities and assist those most in need
	→	←	Uses secretariat to coordinate and mobilize relief assistance for international emergencies, promote cooperation between societies and represent them in the international field
	→	←	Uses field delegations to assist and advise societies with relief operations and development programs, and encourage regional cooperation
	→	←	Sees national organizations as partners
	→	←	Uses national societies to strengthen the capacities of societies worldwide, and ensures that this assistance is sustainable and consistent
	→	←	Guides and supports the development of its member societies
	→	←	Creates the opportunity for member societies to work together
	→	←	Influences the behavior of those working within the Blue Cloud societies, public and private authorities, and members of the

Worksheet 8. Tactics and Counter Tactics			
			communities where Blue Cloud works to promote humanitarianism
	→	←	Leads one of the premier vaccination services Societies
	→	←	Uses rules in relations with national societies
	→	←	Uses policies for detailed direction for the network's humanitarian action in specific areas
	→	←	Uses policies to define boundaries for the conduct of the network and the people working within it
	→	←	Uses permanent policy review process to ensure all member Society and network staff, delegates, and volunteers can access, understand, and implement policies
	→	←	Involves member Societies in establishing and reviewing policies
	→	←	Has policies in the areas of programs and services; health, social welfare, and youth; emergency response; institutional capacity; and human resources
	→	←	Operates according to its Constitution and rules of procedures

Worksheet 9. Core idea

Category	Suggested Metaphors, Images, Analogies, Role Models	Your Metaphors, Images, etc.	Core idea
Military	Machine gun, rifle, tank		
Geographical	River, waterfall, creek		
Plant	Tree, fern, Venus flytrap		
Transportation	Bus, golf cart, car	train	Separate the Freedonian train and guide them onto parallel tracks
Sports	Caddy, gymnastics, football		
Mechanical	Wrench, Allen key, ratchet		
Insects	Mosquito, ant, butterfly	dragonflies	Freedonian societies are like dragonflies in mating season
Animals	Cougar, puma, rhinoceros		
Role models	Princess Diana, Donald Trump, Gandhi		

Worksheet 9. Core idea			
Your own Category: architecture	Your own metaphors: house, skyscraper, wall	wall	Ignore the walls of Freedonian member societies

Worksheet 10. Nature of the Crisis	
Question	Answer (Y or N)
Do you have to change the values?	N
Choices are: Between self-orientation and community orientation? Between materialism and non-materialism?	 Community orientation Non-materialism
Do you have to choose among the values for a priority?	N
Choices are: Self-orientations over materialism or non-materialism Community orientation over materialism or non-materialism Materialism over self-orientation or community orientation Non-materialism over self-orientation or community orientation	
Do you have to change the type of strategy?	Y
Choices are: To direct strategy of action To direct strategy of persuasion To indirect strategy of action To indirect strategy of persuasion	 Y
Do you have to change the core idea?	Y
Do you have to change the categories of tactics?	Y

Worksheet 11. Events Leading Up to Crisis	
Comes into being, founded by a military physician	
Acquires legal status through Freedonian Blue Cloud Act	
Joins International Network early	
Adopts International Network's principles of neutrality	

Worksheet 12. Tactics Before and During the Crisis		
Event	Type	Tactic
Organizes global health improvement program	Planned	Y
Begins national immunization programs in 1947	Planned	Y
Provides immunization for four decades	Planned	Y
Sickens and kill some people with its improperly prepared vaccines	Crisis	N
Welcomes a government inquiry	Coping	Y
Accepts loss of its vaccination programs to the newly created Freedonian vaccine services Association	Coping	Y
Moves forward with its remaining objectives in humanitarianism	Coping	Y
Formulates three strategic pillars of advocacy, capacity building, and crisis intervention	Coping	Y

Worksheet 13. Key Actors	
Number	Key Actors
1	International Network
2	Freedonian Government

Worksheet 14. Key Actors by Tactic Category of Tactic: ______planned_________________		
Tactic	Can Key Actor 1 Affect? (Y or N)	Can Key Actor 2 Affect? (Y or N)
Organizes global health improvement program	Y	Y
Begins national immunization programs in 1947	Y	Y
Provides immunization for four decades	Y	Y

Worksheet 14. Key Actors by Tactic Category of Tactic: ______crisis_________________		
Tactic	Can Key Actor 1 Affect? (Y or N)	Can Key Actor 2 Affect? (Y or N)
Sickens and kill some people with its improperly prepared vaccines	N	N

Worksheet 14. Key Actors by Tactic Category of Tactic: ______coping_________________		
Tactic	Can Key Actor 1 Affect? (Y or N)	Can Key Actor 2 Affect? (Y or N)
Welcomes a government inquiry	Y	Y
Accepts loss of its vaccination programs to the newly created Freedonian vaccine services Association	N	N
Moves forward with its remaining objectives in humanitarianism	Y	N
Formulates three strategic pillars of advocacy, capacity building, and crisis intervention	Y	N

Worksheet 15. Key Rules	
Number	Possible Key Rules
1	Policy of one society per state for International Network
2	Procedures for International Network

Worksheet 16. Key Rules by Tactic Category of Tactic: _____planned________		
Tactic	Can Key Rule 1 Affect? (Y or N)	Can Key Rule 2 Affect? (Y or N)
Organizes global health improvement program	N	Y

Worksheet 16. Key Rules by Tactic Category of Tactic: _____planned________		
Begins national immunization programs in 1947	N	Y
Provides immunization for four decades	N	Y

Worksheet 16. Key Rules by Tactic Category of Tactic: _____crisis________		
Tactic	Can Key Rule 1 Affect? (Y or N)	Can Key Rule 2 Affect? (Y or N)
Sickens and kill some people with its improperly prepared vaccines	N	N

Worksheet 16. Key Rules by Tactic Category of Tactic: _____coping________		
Tactic	Can Key Rule 1 Affect? (Y or N)	Can Key Rule 2 Affect? (Y or N)
Welcomes a government inquiry	N	N
Accepts loss of its vaccination programs to the newly created Freedonian vaccine services Association	Y	Y
Moves forward with its remaining objectives in humanitarianism	Y	N
Formulates three strategic pillars of advocacy, capacity building, and crisis intervention	N	N

Worksheet 17. Key Resources	
Number	Possible Key Resource
1	Expertise developed through operations
2	Money for staff
3	Money for coordination
4	Information on views of member societies

Worksheet 18. Key Resources by Tactic Category of Tactic: planned				
Tactic	Can Key Resource 1 Affect? (Y or N)	Can Key Resource 2 Affect? (Y or N)	Can Key Resource 3 Affect? (Y or N)	Can Key Resource 4 Affect? (Y or N)
Organizes global health improvement program	Y	Y	Y	N
Begins national immunization programs in 1947	Y	Y	N	N
Provides immunization for four decades	Y	Y	N	N

Worksheet 18. Key Resources by Tactic Category of Tactic: crisis				
Tactic	Can Key Resource 1 Affect? (Y or N)	Can Key Resource 2 Affect? (Y or N)	Can Key Resource 3 Affect? (Y or N)	Can Key Resource 4 Affect? (Y or N)
Sickens and kill some people with its improperly prepared vaccines	Y	N	N	N

Worksheet 18. Key Resources by Tactic Category of Tactic: coping				
Tactic	Can Key Resource 1 Affect? (Y or N)	Can Key Resource 2 Affect? (Y or N)	Can Key Resource 3 Affect? (Y or N)	Can Key Resource 4 Affect? (Y or N)
Welcomes a government inquiry	N	N	N	Y
Accepts loss of its vaccination programs to the newly created Freedonian vaccine services Association	N	N	N	Y
Moves forward with its remaining objectives in humanitarianism	Y	Y	Y	Y
Formulates three strategic pillars of advocacy, capacity building, and crisis intervention	Y	Y	N	N

Worksheet 19. Possible Key Factors	
Number	Possible Key Factors
1	Natural disaster
2	COVID-19 pandemic

Worksheet 20. Key Factors by Tactic Category of Tactic: planned		
Tactic	Can Key Factor 1 Affect? (Y or N)	Can Key Factor 2 Affect? (Y or N)
Organizes global health improvement program	Y	Y
Begins national immunization programs in 1947	Y	Y
Provides immunization for four decades	Y	Y

Worksheet 20. Key Factors by Tactic Category of Tactic: crisis		
Tactic	Can Key Factor 1 Affect? (Y or N)	Can Key Factor 2 Affect? (Y or N)
Sickens and kill some people with its improperly prepared vaccines	Y	Y

Worksheet 20. Key Factors by Tactic Category of Tactic: coping		
Tactic	Can Key Factor 1 Affect? (Y or N)	Can Key Factor 2 Affect? (Y or N)
Welcomes a government inquiry	Y	N
Accepts loss of its vaccination programs to the newly created Freedonian vaccine services Association	N	Y
Moves forward with its remaining objectives in humanitarianism	Y	Y
Formulates three strategic pillars of advocacy, capacity building, and crisis intervention	Y	Y

Worksheet 21. Tactical Goal					
Option	Description	Goal	Likelihood of success	Benefits	Costs
1	Accept losing vaccination	Continue its humanitarian work with International Network	75%	Requires negotiations with International Network to retain working relationship	Prestige Fundraising appeal for flagship program
2	Fight losing vaccination	Continue its humanitarian work with International Network	75%	Possibility of retaining full terms of reference guarantees work with International Network	Money to pay for legal challenge Lost opportunities in humanitarian work

Worksheet 22. Tactic Design		
Component \ Option	Option 1: accept losing vaccination program	Option 2: fight losing vaccination program
Time required	2-3 months	2-3 years
Deadline	n/a	n/a
Place	Freedonian	Freedonia
Actor(s)	Freedonian Blue Cloud, Freedonian government, International Network	Freedonian courts, Freedonian lawyers, Freedonian government lawyers

Worksheet 22. Tactic Design		
Action	Negotiations with International Network	Civil proceedings in Freedonian courts
Information needed	Policies and Procedures at International Network	Legal arguments against govt removing vaccination programs from jurisdiction
Collaboration needed from	International Network secretariat and board	n/a
Inaction needed from	n/a	Freedonian Vaccination Services
Other requirements	n/a	n/a

Worksheet 23. Options by Node	
Options by Node	
Node	Option
Freedonian government creates new vaccination agency	Accept losing vaccination programs

Worksheet 24. List of Individual Tactics, Option 1		
Number	Tactic	Description
1	Acceptance	Announce acceptance
2	Preparation and separation	Prepare for loss of vaccination programs, complete separation of staff
3	Administrative review	Review policies, procedures, budget, charter of Freedonian Blue Cloud and amend as appropriate
4	IN Process	Consult with International Network secretariat and board, follow procedures given, secure approval, make changes as necessary

Worksheet 25. Design of Individual Tactics Tactic: acceptance				
Component	Tactic 1	Tactic 2	Tactic 3	Tactic 4
Action	Announce acceptance	Preparation for loss of programs	Administrative review	IN process
Actor	Freedonian Blue Cloud board	Freedonian Blue Cloud Board	Freedonian Blue Cloud	Freedonian Blue Cloud board
Deadline	n/a	As given by Freedonian government	n/a	n/a
Location	Freedonia	Freedonia	Freedonia	Gubbio, Italy
Information needed	How to make announcement known to public	Budget requirements for two entities	Budget and staff for smaller organization	Policies, procedures, charter for IN, willingness of

Worksheet 25. Design of Individual Tactics Tactic: acceptance				
				IN Board to consider request
Time needed	2 weeks	Several months	Several months	Several months
Material Needed	Means of communication	New offices and supplies	Offices and supplies	Offices and supplies, means of communication and travel
Important Rules	Informing staff first	New and amended charters, policies, procedures	Charter, policies	Policies, procedures for IN Board and secretariat
Important People	Staff, Freedonian government, Freedonian public	Both boards, both staff members	Board and staff members for Freedonian Blue Cloud	IN secretariat, IN Board, Freedonian Blue Cloud staff

Chapter 7

Two International Organizations Interact

This is the story of the relations between the Organization for Preventing Cognitive Impairment (OPCI) and the World Mental Health Organization (WMHO).

OPCI

OPCI's key role is to build and strengthen national associations throughout the world, so they are better able to meet the needs of people with cognitive impairment and their families. OPCI's goals include the support and the strengthening of member associations in their activities; the creation and support of new associations; collaboration with the World Mental Health Organization and other international organizations with similar interests; and increasing public and political awareness at national and international level; and the support of research. OPCI is governed by a 20-member council, including an executive committee and a representative from each full member organization. The council meets once a year during the annual international conference. OPCI also has a medical and scientific advisory panel whose role is to provide expert advice when necessary and act as international ambassadors for OPCI. Each of the member associations is the national cognitive impairment association in its own country. Each member association supports people with cognitive impairment and their families. Most of the member associations are in developing countries where health and social services are limited: the association may be the only support available.

OPCI strengthens the work of its members through an annual international conference, the OPCI Training Center, a World Cognitive Impairment Day, and the support of research and public education and information. The annual international conference is hosted by a different member each year. The conference is an opportunity to bring everyone with an interest in cognitive impairment to share and learn from each other: staff and volunteers of associations from around the world, families, people living with cognitive impairment themselves, clinicians, interested professionals, and scientists. The OPCI Training Center helps associations to help themselves: it provides a series of workshops designed to build organizational capacity by focusing on the fundamental issues of setting up and running an association. World Cognitive Impairment Day is a day on which member associations concentrate their efforts on raising awareness about the estimated 18 million people around the world who currently have cognitive impairment. Each year a special theme is selected, about which OPCI prepares and distributes promotional materials around the world. OPCI financially supports the Cognitive Impairment Group: this network is made up of 200 active researchers from 42 developing countries who are studying the prevalence and impact of cognitive impairment in communities where it has not been studied before. Finally, OPCI produces a range of publications - a newsletter, fact sheets as necessary, booklets, and a video for primary care doctors about cognitive impairment. Most materials are available in French, Spanish and English. Materials for caregivers are available in Chinese, Russian, German, Hindi, Arabic and Portuguese. Information in other languages is also available locally. Publications can be downloaded free.

WORLD MENTAL HEALTH ORGANIZATION (WMHO)

The World Mental Health Organization is a specialized agency for mental health. It was established, along with the World Health Organization, in 1948. The WMHO's objective, as set out in its constitution, is the attainment by all peoples of the highest possible level of mental health. Mental health is defined as a state of complete mental and social well-being and not merely the absence of disease or infirmity. The WMHO is governed by the 192 Member States through the General Mental Health Assembly. This assembly is composed of representatives from WMHO's member states. The main tasks of the assembly are to approve the WMHO programs and budget, and to decide major policy questions.

The Secretariat is headed by the Director-General, who is nominated by the Executive Board and elected by Member States for a period of five years. The Secretariat is staffed by mental health professionals, other experts and support staff working at headquarters in Geneva, in the six regional offices and in countries. WMHO's regional offices are in Brazzaville for Africa, Bucharest for Europe, Singapore for South-East Asia, Washington for the Americas, Beirut for the Eastern Mediterranean, and Kuala Lumpur for the Western Pacific. In carrying out its activities, WMHO's secretariat focuses on: articulating consistent, ethical and evidence-based policy and advocacy positions; managing information by assessing trends and comparing performance; setting the agenda for, and stimulating research and development; catalyzing change through technical and policy support, in ways that stimulate cooperation and action and help to build sustainable national and inter-country capacity; negotiating and sustaining national and global partnerships; setting, validating, monitoring and pursuing the proper implementation of norms and standards; and stimulating the development and testing of new technologies, tools and guidelines for control, risk reduction, health care management, and service delivery for mental health.

The WMHO constitution states that the enjoyment of the highest attainable standard of mental health is one of the fundamental rights of every human being without distinction of race, religion, politics, economic or social condition. It also states that the achievement of any state in the promotion and protection of mental health is of value to all. Unequal development in different countries in the promotion of mental health and the prevention of mental illness and impairment is a common issue. The healthy mental development of the child is of basic importance. Governments all have a responsibility for the mental health of their peoples which can be fulfilled only by the provision of adequate mental health and social measures.

The four directions for the WMHO are: reducing excess morbidity, disability and even mortality, especially in poor and marginalized populations; reducing risk factors to mental health that arise from environmental, economic, social and behavioral causes; developing mental health systems that equitably improve outcomes, respond to people's legitimate demands, and are financially fair; and framing and enabling policy and creating an institutional environment for the mental health sector, and promoting an effective mental health dimension to social, economic, environmental and development policy. One of the main functions of the WMHO is to direct and coordinate an international mental health approach. The WMHO consults and cooperates with nongovern-mental organizations (NGOs), including the OPCI. WMHO's collaboration with the OPCI seeks to promote its own policies, strategies, and programs; to collaborate with various WMHO programs in jointly agreed activities to implement these strategies; and to play an appropriate role in harmonizing inter-sectoral interests. The WMHO's slogan is 'Mental health for all'.

OPCI/WMHO Interactions

Collaboration was affected in practice by the COVID pandemic, if not in goals or philosophy. In its interactions with the WMHO, the OPCI is responsible for implementing the mutually agreed program of collaboration and informs the WMHO as soon as possible if for any reason they are unable to fulfill their part of the agreement. OPCI uses the opportunities available to them through their normal work to disseminate information on WMHO policies and programs. OPCI collaborates individually or collectively in

WMHO programs to further mental-health-for-all goals. OPCI individually or collectively collaborates with the member states of the WMHO where their activities are based in the implementation of the national/regional/global health-for-all strategies. Generally, in its interactions with NGOs, the WMHO recognizes only official relations with those NGOs which meet the criteria described in its principles. The establishment of relations with NGOs is an evolving process. First contacts include exchanges of information and reciprocal participation in technical meetings on an ad hoc basis. Next, collaboration can proceed for two years, starting with an exchange of letters setting out the agreed basis for it. This is assessed and may continue for another two years or result in an application to the WMHO board for a long-term and closer relationship. For the board to admit an organization, that organization's main area of competence must fall within the purview of WMHO, and it must center on development work in mental health or mental health-related fields without a commercial or profit-making nature.

OPCI meets the criteria for official relations with WMHO. OPCI is international in its structure and scope, and it represents a substantial proportion of the persons globally organized for the purpose of participating in the field of interest in which it operates. OPCI has a constitution, an established headquarters, a directing or governing body, an administrative structure at various levels of action, and authority to speak for its members through its authorized representatives. Its members exercise voting rights in relation to its policies or action. OPCI has also completed over two years of working relations. The procedure for admitting OPCI into official relations with WMHO is specific. OPCI's application should normally reach WMHO headquarters not later than the end of July, to be considered by the Executive Board in January of the following year. It needs to specify a structured plan for collaborative activities agreed upon by the organization and WMHO. OPCI has already obtained the endorsements of the WMHO Regional Director and the government of the US, the site of its headquarters. It was transmitted to Board members by the Secretariat two months in advance of the session at which its application will be considered.

The Board can decide whether an organization such as OPCI is to be admitted into official relations with WMHO. If not, a re-application from an NGO would not normally be considered until two years have elapsed. The Director-General then informs the organization of the Board's decision on its application. The Director-General maintains a list of the organizations admitted into official relations, and this list and any amendments are be circulated to the Members of WMHO. A plan for collaboration based on mutually agreed objectives and outlining activities for the coming three-year period formed the basis of official relations between WMHO and OPCI. This plan is transmitted to the WMHO regional offices to encourage closer collaboration at regional level as appropriate.

Once OPCI is admitted, the board reviews collaboration with the OPCI every three years. There are several privileges conferred by official relationship with the WMHO. One is the right to appoint a representative to participate, without right of vote, in the WMHO's meetings or in those of the committees and conferences convened under its authority. A second is the access to non-confidential documentation. A third is the right to submit a memorandum to the Director-General, which might be placed on the agenda of the General Mental Health Assembly.

This semi-fictional case study presents the variant where, rather than a crisis, an opportunity presents itself: the application for formal relations from OPCI.

Worksheet 1. Strategy		
Issue/Problem	Poor mental health in the nations of the world	
Goal	Improve mental health	
Core idea (metaphor, slogan, etc.)	'Mental health for all"	
Tactics (actions or bundles of actions)	1	reducing excess morbidity, disability and even mortality, especially in poor and marginalized populations
	2	reducing risk factors to mental health that arise from environmental, economic, social, and behavioral cause
	3	developing mental health systems that equitably improve outcomes, respond to people's legitimate demands, and are financially fair
	4	framing an enabling policy and creating an institutional environment for the mental health sector, and promoting an

Worksheet 1. Strategy		
		effective mental health dimension to social, economic, environmental and development policy

Worksheet 2. Key Actors	
All Actors	Can this actor affect your achieving the goal? (Yes or No)
Public in OPCI member organizations' countries	Y
OPCI council	Y
OPCI executive committee	Y
OPCI representatives from member organizations	Y
OPCI medical and scientific advisory panel	Y
People with cognitive impairment	Y
Families of cognitively impaired people	Y
OPCI staff	Y
OPCI volunteers	Y
OPCI member organizations staff	Y
OPCI member organizations volunteers	Y
Clinicians	Y
Professionals	Y
Scientists	Y
OPCI Training Center	Y
WMHO's regional offices	Y
WMHO	Y
Every human being	N
Governments	Y
Poor and marginalized populations	Y
Nongovernmental organizations (NGOs)	Y
OPCI	Y
Member states of the WMHO	Y
WMHO board	Y
Member organizations of OPCI	Y
OPCI headquarters	Y
OPCI board	Y
WMHO headquarters	Y
WMHO regional director	Y
US government	Y
WMHO secretariat	Y
WMHO director-general	Y
OPCI representative to WMHO	Y
WMHO General Mental Health Assembly	Y

Worksheet 3. An Actor's Actions and Tactics		
Actor: WMHO		
Time/Date	Action	Is this a tactic? (Yes or No)
1948	Establishes itself	Y
	Writes constitution	Y
	Creates assembly	Y
	Creates board	Y
	Elects director-general	Y
	Hires staff	Y
	Creates secretariat	Y
	Provides secretariat with focus	Y
	Adopts highest standard of mental health as fundamental right of every human being without distinction	Y
	Considers the healthy mental development of the child of basic importance	Y
	States governments have a responsibility for the mental health of their peoples	Y
	Identifies its four key directions	Y
	Directs and coordinates international mental health approach	Y
	Cooperates with NGOs	Y
	Receives information from NGOS with formal or informal relations	Y
	Receives information from OPCI	Y
	Recognizes official relations only with those NGOs which meet its principles	Y
	Establishes relations with NGOs	Y
	Enters two-year relations with NGOs	Y
	Reviews relations with NGOs periodically	Y
	Admits NGOs to formal relations	Y
	Entertains applications from NGOs	Y
	Affords three privileges to member NGOs	Y

Worksheet 4. Resources a Strategy Can Draw On			
Resource	Do you have enough? (Y or N)	Is this a 'nice to have?'	Is this a 'must have'?
Money for staff	N		Y
Methods of transportation for meetings	N		Y
Money for offices and supplies	N		Y
Methods of communication	Y		Y
Information on major policy questions	N		Y

Worksheet 4. Resources a Strategy Can Draw On			
Information on laws and policies on mental health around the world	N		Y
Information on trends	N		Y
Information on performance	N		Y
Information on norms and standards of mental health	N		Y
Information on guidelines for control of mental health	N		Y
Information on risk reduction for mental health	N		Y
Information on national and global capacity	N		Y
Information on mental health care management	N		Y
Information on mental health service delivery	N		Y
Information in each country on promotion of mental health	N		Y
Information in each country on prevention of mental illness or impairment	N		Y
Information on mental health of children in each country	N		Y
Information in each country of excess morbidity, disability, and mortality	N		Y
Information on risk factors from environmental, economic, social, and behavioral causes	N		Y
Information on member and prospective member organizations	N		Y
Time to work with NGOs	N		Y
Time to consider applications from NGOs	Y		Y
Time for meetings	Y		Y
Time for decisions	N		Y
Time for preparation for meetings	N		Y

Worksheet 5. What you can and cannot do		
Rule	Does this rule help you reach your goal?	Does breaking this rule guarantee your failure?
Constitution	Y	N
Policies	Y	N
Procedures	Y	N
Decisions by assembly	Y	N
Decisions by board	Y	N
Laws in host nations for regional offices	N	Y
Laws in headquarter host nation	N	Y
Standards of mental health in member stations	N	Y

Worksheet 5. What you can and cannot do		
Health regulations for mental health in member nations	N	Y

Worksheet 6. Factors Outside Your Control			
Desired Strategic Outcome:			
Factors that help		Factors that do not help	
	→	←	Natural disaster
	→	←	COVID-19 pandemic

Worksheet 7. Do or Die Moments	
Goal: mental health for all	
Steps to Goal	Problem 1
Establishes itself ▼	
Writes constitution ▼	
Creates assembly ▼	
Creates board ▼	
Elects director-general ▼	
Hires staff ▼	
Creates secretariat ▼	
Provides secretariat with focus ▼	
Adopts highest standard of mental health as fundamental right of every human being without distinction ▼	
Considers the healthy mental development of the child of basic importance ▼	
States governments have a responsibility for the mental health of their peoples ▼	
Identifies its four key directions ▼	
Directs and coordinates international mental health approach ▼	
Cooperates with NGOs ▼	

Worksheet 7. Do or Die Moments	
Receives information from NGOS with formal or informal relations ▼	
Recognizes official relations only with those NGOs which meet its principles ▼	
Establishes relations with NGOs ▼	
Enters two-year relations with NGOs ▼	
Reviews relations with NGOs periodically ▼	
Admits NGOs to formal relations ▼	
Entertains applications from NGOs ▼	
Affords three privileges to member NGOs ▼	Receives information from OPCI ▼

Use as many columns or rows as you need. When you are done:
BOLD or CIRCLE EACH DO-OR-DIE MOMENT.

Worksheet 8. Tactics and Counter Tactics			
Your Goal: mental health for all		Their Goal: have a formal relationship with WMHO	
Your Tactics		Their Countervailing Tactics	
Establishes itself	→	←	Identified key role
Writes constitution	→	←	Supports member associations
Creates assembly	→	←	Collaborates with WMHO
Creates board	→	←	Increases public awareness at national and international level
Elects director-general	→	←	Increases political awareness at national and international level
Hires staff	→	←	Has executive meetings once a year
Creates secretariat	→	←	Receives advice from medical and scientific advisory panel
Provides secretariat with focus	→	←	Holds annual international conference
Adopts highest standard of mental health as fundamental right of	→	←	Educates public through World Cognitive Impairment day

Worksheet 8. Tactics and Counter Tactics			
every human being without distinction			
Considers the healthy mental development of the child of basic importance	→	←	Supports research
States governments have a responsibility for the mental health of their peoples	→	←	Supports public education and information
Identifies its four key directions	→	←	Implements program of collaboration with WMHO
Directs and coordinates international mental health approach	→	←	Informs WMHO if they cannot fulfill obligations
Cooperates with NGOs	→	←	Provides workshops designed to build organizational capacity in member organization
Receives information from NGOS with formal or informal relations	→	←	Produces multilingual publications
Recognizes official relations only with those NGOs which meet its principles	→	←	Uses its own work opportunities to disseminate information on WMHO policies and programs
Establishes relations with NGOs	→	←	Collaborates individually or collectively in WMHO programs to further health-for-all goals
Enters two-year relations with NGOs	→	←	Collaborates with WMHO member states in national/regional/global mental health-for-all strategies
Reviews relations with NGOs periodically	→	←	Represents a substantial proportion of the persons globally organized in its field of interest
Admits NGOs to formal relations	→	←	Has voting members
Entertains applications from NGOs	→	←	Applies to WMHO
Affords three privileges to member NGOs	→	←	Provides a structured plan for collaborative activities with WMHO
Receives information from OPCI	→	←	Obtains the endorsements of the WMHO Regional Director and the government of the US

Worksheet 9. Core idea			
Category	Suggested Metaphors, Images, Analogies, Role Models	Your Metaphors, Images, etc.	Core idea
Military	Machine gun, rifle, tank	Machine gun	WMHO will riddle mental illness with holes
Geographical	River, waterfall, creek	Ocean	WMHO will bring an ocean of mental health to the world
Plant	Tree, fern, Venus flytrap	Venus flytrap	WMHO will trap and digest mental illness worldwide
Transportation	Bus, golf cart, car		
Sports	Caddy, gymnastics, football		
Mechanical	Wrench, Allen key, ratchet		
Insects	Mosquito, ant, butterfly		
Animals	Cougar, puma, rhinoceros	Hippopotamus	WMHO trample mental illness wherever it finds it
Role models	Princess Diana, Donald Trump, Gandhi		
Your own Category:	Your own metaphors:		

Worksheet 10. Nature of the Crisis	
Question	Answer (Y or N)
Do you have to change the values?	N
Choices are: Between self-orientation and community orientation? Between materialism and non-materialism?	
Do you have to choose among the values for a priority?	N
Choices are: Self-orientations over materialism or non-materialism Community orientation over materialism or non-materialism Materialism over self-orientation or community orientation Non-materialism over self-orientation or community orientation	
Do you have to change the type of strategy?	N
Choices are: To direct strategy of action To direct strategy of persuasion To indirect strategy of action To indirect strategy of persuasion	
Do you have to change the core idea?	N
Do you have to change the categories of tactics?	

Worksheet 11. Events Leading Up to Crisis	
Establishes itself	
Writes constitution	
Creates assembly	
Creates board	
Elects director-general	
Hires staff	
Creates secretariat	
Provides secretariat with focus	
Adopts highest standard of mental health as fundamental right of every human being without distinction	
Considers the healthy mental development of the child of basic importance	
States governments have a responsibility for the mental health of their peoples	
Identifies its four key directions	
Directs and coordinates international mental health approach	
Cooperates with NGOs	
Receives information from NGOS with formal or informal relations	
Recognizes official relations only with those NGOs which meet its principles	
Establishes relations with NGOs	
Enters two-year relations with NGOs	
Reviews relations with NGOs periodically	
Admits NGOs to formal relations	
Entertains applications from NGOs	
Affords three privileges to member NGOs	
Receives information from OPCI	
	Receives application from OPCI

Worksheet 12. Tactics Before and During the Crisis		
Event	Type	Tactic
Establishes itself	Planned	Y
Writes constitution	Planned	Y
Creates assembly	Planned	Y
Creates board	Planned	Y
Elects director-general	Planned	Y
Hires staff	Planned	Y

Worksheet 12. Tactics Before and During the Crisis		
Creates secretariat	Planned	Y
Provides secretariat with focus	Planned	Y
Adopts highest standard of mental health as fundamental right of every human being without distinction	Planned	Y
Considers the healthy mental development of the child of basic importance	Planned	Y
States governments have a responsibility for the mental health of their peoples	Planned	Y
Identifies its four key directions	Planned	Y
Directs and coordinates international mental health approach	Planned	Y
Cooperates with NGOs	Planned	Y
Receives information from NGOS with formal or informal relations	Planned	Y
Recognizes official relations only with those NGOs which meet its principles	Planned	Y
Establishes relations with NGOs	Planned	Y
Enters two-year relations with NGOs	Planned	Y
Reviews relations with NGOs periodically	Planned	Y
Admits NGOs to formal relations	Planned	Y
Entertains applications from NGOs	Planned	Y
Affords three privileges to member NGOs	Planned	Y
Receives information from OPCI	Planned	Y

Worksheet 12. Tactics Before and During the Crisis		
Event	Type	Tactic
Receives application from OPCI	crisis	Y

Worksheet 13. Key Actors	
Number	Key Actors
1	OPCI

Worksheet 14. Key Actors by Tactic Category of Tactic: ____planned__________________	
Tactic	Can Key Actor 1 Affect? (Y or N)
Establishes itself	N
Writes constitution	N
Creates assembly	N
Creates board	N
Elects director-general	N
Hires staff	N
Creates secretariat	N
Provides secretariat with focus	N

Worksheet 14. Key Actors by Tactic Category of Tactic: ____planned___________________	
Adopts highest standard of mental health as fundamental right of every human being without distinction	N
Considers the healthy mental development of the child of basic importance	N
States governments have a responsibility for the mental health of their peoples	N
Identifies its four key directions	N
Directs and coordinates international mental health approach	N
Cooperates with NGOs	Y
Receives information from NGOS with formal or informal relations	Y
Recognizes official relations only with those NGOs which meet its principles	Y
Establishes relations with NGOs	Y
Enters two-year relations with NGOs	Y
Reviews relations with NGOs periodically	Y
Admits NGOs to formal relations	Y
Entertains applications from NGOs	Y
Affords three privileges to member NGOs	Y
Receives information from OPCI	Y

Worksheet 14. Key Actors by Tactic Category of Tactic: ____crisis___________________	
Tactic	Can Key Actor 1 Affect? (Y or N)
Receives OPCI application	Y

Worksheet 15. Key Rules	
Number	Possible Key Rules
1	Policies
2	Procedures
3	Decisions by board

Worksheet 16. Key Rules by Tactic Category of Tactic: __planned___________			
Tactic	Can Key Rule 1 Affect? (Y or N)	Can Key Rule 2 Affect? (Y or N)	Can Key Rule 3 Affect? (Y or N)
Establishes itself	N	N	N
Writes constitution	N	N	N
Creates assembly	Y	Y	N
Creates board	Y	Y	N
Elects director-general	Y	Y	Y
Hires staff	Y	Y	Y
Creates secretariat	Y	Y	Y

Worksheet 16. Key Rules by Tactic Category of Tactic: __planned___________			
Provides secretariat with focus	Y	Y	Y
Adopts highest standard of mental health as fundamental right of every human being without distinction	Y	Y	Y
Considers the healthy mental development of the child of basic importance	Y	Y	Y
States governments have a responsibility for the mental health of their peoples	Y	Y	Y
Identifies its four key directions	Y	Y	Y
Directs and coordinates international mental health approach	Y	Y	Y
Cooperates with NGOs	Y	Y	Y
Receives information from NGOS with formal or informal relations	Y	Y	Y
Recognizes official relations only with those NGOs which meet its principles	Y	Y	Y
Establishes relations with NGOs	Y	Y	Y
Enters two-year relations with NGOs	Y	Y	Y
Reviews relations with NGOs periodically	Y	Y	Y
Admits NGOs to formal relations	Y	Y	Y
Entertains applications from NGOs	Y	Y	Y
Affords three privileges to member NGOs	Y	Y	Y
Receives information from OPCI	Y	Y	Y

Worksheet 16. Key Rules by Tactic Category of Tactic: __crisis___________			
Tactic	Can Key Rule 1 Affect? (Y or N)	Can Key Rule 2 Affect? (Y or N)	Can Key Rule 3 Affect? (Y or N)
Receives OPCI application	Y	Y	Y

Worksheet 17. Key Resources	
Number	Possible Key Resource
1	Information in each country on promotion of mental health
2	Information in each country on prevention of mental illness or impairment
3	Information on member and prospective member organizations
4	Time to work with NGOs
5	Time to consider applications from NGOs

Worksheet 18. Key Resources by Tactic Category of Tactic: ____planned_________					
Tactic	Can Key Resource 1 Affect? (Y or N)	Can Key Resource 2 Affect? (Y or N)	Can Key Resource 3 Affect? (Y or N)	Can Key Resource 4 Affect? (Y or N)	Can Key Resource 5 Affect? (Y or N)
Establishes itself	N	N	N	N	N
Writes constitution	N	N	N	N	N
Creates assembly	N	N	N	N	N
Creates board	N	N	N	N	N
Elects director-general	N	N	N	N	N
Hires staff	N	N	N	N	N
Creates secretariat	N	N	N	N	N
Provides secretariat with focus	N	N	N	N	N
Adopts highest standard of mental health as fundamental right of every human being without distinction	N	N	N	N	N
Considers the healthy mental development of the child of basic importance	N	N	N	N	N
States governments have a responsibility for the mental health of their peoples	N	N	N	N	N
Identifies its four key directions	N	N	N	N	N
Directs and coordinates international mental health approach	N	N	N	N	N
Cooperates with NGOs	Y	Y	Y	Y	Y
Receives information from NGOS with formal or informal relations	Y	Y	Y	Y	Y
Recognizes official relations only with	Y	Y	Y	Y	Y

Worksheet 18. Key Resources by Tactic Category of Tactic: ____planned_________					
those NGOs which meet its principles					
Establishes relations with NGOs	Y	Y	Y	Y	Y
Enters two-year relations with NGOs	Y	Y	Y	Y	Y
Reviews relations with NGOs periodically	Y	Y	Y	Y	Y
Admits NGOs to formal relations	Y	Y	Y	Y	Y
Entertains applications from NGOs	Y	Y	Y	Y	Y
Affords three privileges to member NGOs	Y	Y	Y	Y	Y
Receives information from OPCI	Y	Y	Y	Y	Y

Worksheet 18. Key Resources by Tactic Category of Tactic: ______crisis_______					
Tactic	Can Key Resource 1 Affect? (Y or N)	Can Key Resource 2 Affect? (Y or N)	Can Key Resource 3 Affect? (Y or N)	Can Key Resource 4 Affect? (Y or N)	Can Key Resource 5 Affect? (Y or N)
Receives OPCI application	Y	Y	Y	Y	Y

Worksheet 19. Possible Key Factors	
Number	Possible Key Factors
1	Natural disaster
2	COVID-19 pandemic

Worksheet 20. Key Factors by Tactic Category of Tactic: planned		
Tactic	Can Key Factor 1 Affect? (Y or N)	Can Key Factor 2 Affect? (Y or N)
Establishes itself	Y	Y
Writes constitution	Y	Y
Creates assembly	Y	Y
Creates board	Y	Y

Worksheet 20. Key Factors by Tactic Category of Tactic: planned		
Elects director-general	Y	Y
Hires staff	Y	Y
Creates secretariat	Y	Y
Provides secretariat with focus	Y	Y
Adopts highest standard of mental health as fundamental right of every human being without distinction	Y	Y
Considers the healthy mental development of the child of basic importance	Y	Y
States governments have a responsibility for the mental health of their peoples	Y	Y
Identifies its four key directions	Y	Y
Directs and coordinates international mental health approach	Y	Y
Cooperates with NGOs	Y	Y
Receives information from NGOS with formal or informal relations	Y	Y
Recognizes official relations only with those NGOs which meet its principles	Y	Y
Establishes relations with NGOs	Y	Y
Enters two-year relations with NGOs	Y	Y
Reviews relations with NGOs periodically	Y	Y
Admits NGOs to formal relations	Y	Y
Entertains applications from NGOs	Y	Y
Affords three privileges to member NGOs	Y	Y
Receives information from OPCI	Y	Y

Worksheet 20. Key Factors by Tactic Category of Tactic:		
Tactic	Can Key Factor 1 Affect? (Y or N)	Can Key Factor 2 Affect? (Y or N)
Receives OPCI application	Y	Y

Worksheet 21. Tactical Goal					
Opti-on	Descrip-tion	Goal	Likelihood of success	Benefits	Costs
1	Accepts application	Work with another NGO to further goals	100%	Expands people working towards WMHO goals	May dampen enthusiasm for developing capacity
2	Rejects application	Work with an NGO to reach the standards of long-term association	100%	Greater incentive for NGO to develop capacity	May dampen enthusiasm for collaborating with WMHO

Worksheet 22. Tactic Design		
Option / Component	Option 1: accept application	Option 2: reject application
Time required	3 months	3 months
Deadline	n/a	n/a
Place	Geneva	Geneva
Actor(s)	Director general, secretariat, board	Director general, secretariat, board
Action	Present documentation, hold meeting, make decision, communicate decision	Present documentation, hold meeting, make decision, communicate decision
Information needed	How OPCI meets WMHO criteria	How OPCI meets WMHO criteria
Collaboration needed from	OPCI board, executive director, staff	OPCI board, executive director, staff
Inaction needed from	n/a	n/a
Other requirements	n/a	n/a

Worksheet 23. Options by Node	
Options by Node	
Node	Option
Receives OPCI application	Accept
	Reject

Worksheet 24. List of Individual Tactics, Option accept		
Number	Tactic	Description
1	Present documentation	Obtain from applicant document on how it meets the criteria for formal relations with WMHO
2	Hold meeting	Prepare meeting documentation, submit it to members, set meeting agenda, organize logistics of meeting, hold meeting
3	Make decision	Consider application, discuss whether it meets criteria
4	Communicate decision	Write letter to applicant

Worksheet 24. List of Individual Tactics, Option reject		
Number	Tactic	Description
1	Present documentation	Obtain from applicant document on how it meets the criteria for formal relations with WMHO
2	Hold meeting	Prepare meeting documentation, submit it to members, set meeting agenda, organize logistics of meeting, hold meeting
3	Make decision	Consider application, discuss whether it meets criteria, provide reasons for decision, outline work yet to be done
4	Communicate decision	Write letter to applicant

In this case study, the actions to be taken are similar for both options.

Worksheet 25. Design of Individual Tactics
Tactic: accept

Component	Tactic 1	Tactic 2	Tactic 3	Tactic 4
Action	Obtain from applicant document on how it meets the criteria for formal relations with WMHO	Prepare meeting documentation, submit it to members, set meeting agenda, organize logistics of meeting, hold meeting	Consider application, discuss whether it meets criteria	Write letter to applicant
Actor	Director general	Director general	WMHO board members	Director general
Deadline	Next board meeting	Next board meeting	End of board meeting	n/a
Location	Geneva	Geneva	Geneva	Geneva
Information needed	How applicant meets criteria How to communicate with applicant	Address for each board member	How applicant meets criteria	Address for applicant
Time needed	1 month	1 month	Several hours	1 month
Material needed	Office space and supplies, staff support	Office space and supplies, staff support	Office space and supplies, staff support, meeting space	Office space and supplies, staff support
Important Rules	WMHO constitution	WMHO constitution	WMHO constitution	WMHO constitution
Important People	OPCI executive director and staff	WMHO board members	WMHO board members	WMHO staff

Worksheet 25. Design of Individual Tactics
Tactic: reject

Component	Tactic 1	Tactic 2	Tactic 3	Tactic 4
Action	Obtain from applicant document on how it meets the criteria for formal relations with WMHO	Prepare meeting documentation, submit it to members, set meeting agenda, organize logistics of meeting, hold meeting	Consider application, discuss whether it meets criteria, provide reasons for decision, outlines work yet to be done by NGO	Write letter to applicant

Worksheet 25. Design of Individual Tactics Tactic: reject				
Actor	Director general	Director general	WMHO board members	Director general
Deadline	Next board meeting	Next board meeting	End of board meeting	n/a
Location	Geneva	Geneva	Geneva	Geneva
Information needed	How applicant meets criteria How to communicate with applicant	Address for each board member	How applicant meets criteria	Address for applicant
Time needed	1 month	1 month	Several hours	1 month
Material needed	Office space and supplies, staff support	Office space and supplies, staff support	Office space and supplies, staff support, meeting space	Office space and supplies, staff support
Important Rules	WMHO constitution	WMHO constitution	WMHO constitution	WMHO constitution
Important People	OPCI executive director and staff	WMHO board members	WMHO board members	WMHO staff

Chapter 8

AN INFRANATIONAL GROUP ENTERTAINS MULTILATERAL RELATIONS

In 1971, a group of young Italian nurses starts Infermiere in volo (IV). IV is an international humanitarian aid organization that aims to rebuild health structures to acceptable levels where they have been destroyed by war, natural disaster, or colonial or authoritarian governments. IV provides emergency medical assistance to populations in danger in more than 100 countries. In countries where health structures are insufficient or even non-existent, IV collaborates with local health authorities. IV also works toward the rehabilitation of hospitals and clinics, establishes vaccination programs and water and sanitation projects. IV works in remote or isolated health care centers, slums, and rural settings. IV provides training of local personnel. It chooses to operate in areas of wars, conflict, and natural or man-made disasters. IV provides a broad range of health services around the world, raises awareness, and develops logistical expertise under the banner of its slogan, "Health without borders".

In 1972, IV's first mission in response to a natural disaster was to the Nicaraguan earthquake. In 1974, Hurricane Fifi hit Honduras, resulting in the first long-term medical assistance mission. In 1976, the civil war in Lebanon presented IV with its first major war mission. For seven months, 70 doctors and nurses took turns in a Beirut hospital. Between 1979 and

1986, wars and refugee crises spread throughout Africa and Asia, and IV set up refugee programs. In the 1979 Soviet invasion of Afghanistan, IV teams worked clandestinely with the Afghan resistance fighters caring for the civilian population. When 1980 brought drought and civil war to Somalia, IV sets up its first nutritional programs in the refugee camps of Kenya. When Communism and Communist societies collapsed starting in 1989, IV set up health programs. The 1991 Kurdish refugee crisis in northern Iraq meant that IV undertook its largest ever emergency relief operations. Between 1993 and 1995, civil war in Burundi and genocide in Rwanda caused complex humanitarian emergencies, for which large numbers of IV volunteers were deployed. IV brought aid inside Chechnya and to the refugee camps of neighboring countries. During a 1996 meningitis outbreak in Nigeria: IV vaccinated millions of people.

Health Services

IV provides primary health care, performs surgery, rehabilitates hospitals and clinics, runs nutrition and sanitation programs, trains local medical personnel, and provides mental health care. Through longer-term programs, it treats chronic diseases such as tuberculosis, malaria, sleeping sickness, and AIDS; assists with the medical and psychological problems of marginalized populations including street children and ethnic minorities; and brings health care to remote, isolated areas where resources and training are limited. Each year, more than 2,500 volunteer doctors, nurses, other medical professionals, logistics experts, water and sanitation engineers, and administrators join 15 000 locally hired staff in over 80 countries.

Raising Awareness

In carrying out humanitarian assistance, IV raises awareness of crisis situations, acting as a witness and speaking out, either in private or in public about the plight of populations in danger. By doing so, IV alleviates human suffering, protects life and health, and restores and ensures respect for the human beings and their fundamental human rights. Only a small percentage of the populations that find themselves in a situation of danger gain the attention of the media. IV teams travel to little-known places to assist them. Whenever possible, volunteers give interviews and make presentations. Offices worldwide facilitate the organization of gatherings, for individuals and groups who want to speak in their home communities. IV also mounts exhibitions and releases publications. Whether testifying at the United Nations or conducting an educational campaign aimed at schoolchildren, the organization works to raise awareness of the plight of the populations it serves. The organization launched public education projects to raise awareness of the trauma faced by children in a war zone, the devastation caused by malnutrition, and the plight of refugees. All IV volunteers are expected to respect the principles of their constitution as well as their own professional ethics. They are not, however, held to the laws of the countries in which they operate if they find them contrary to the principles of the IV constitution. It is part of IV's work to address any violations of basic human rights encountered by field teams, violations perpetrated or sustained by political actors. It does so by confronting the responsible actors themselves, by putting pressure on them through mobilization of the international community and by issuing information publicly. IV maintains neutrality and independence from individual governments and raises most of its funds directly from the public. Typically, there are two education campaigns underway at any given time.

Logistical Capacity

At the onset of emergencies such as COVID-19, teams arrive at a project site with prepackaged medical kits so they can begin working immediately. Custom-designed by IV for specific field situations, geographic conditions, and climates, a kit may contain a complete surgical theater, for example, or all the supplies needed to treat hundreds of cholera patients. IV kits have been replicated by relief organizations worldwide. To maximize its responsiveness to emergency situations, IV maintains four logistical centers based in Europe and East Africa and stocks of emergency materials stored in Central America and East Asia. They purchase, test, and store equipment including vehicles, communications material, power supplies, water-processing facilities, and nutritional supplements. Within 24 hours, planes can be loaded with essential equipment and flown into crisis areas. IV has also developed handbooks for use in the field covering many aspects of relief work, from essential drugs to water and sanitation. These guidelines have been translated into several languages and are used by many other relief organizations. Specialized training of field volunteers is an essential part of the organization's effectiveness: IV offers training programs to an estimated 1 000 participants every year.

GOVERNANCE AND ORGANIZATION

IV has sections in 18 countries. Five of these sections are considered operational, meaning that they directly control field projects—deciding when, where, and what medical relief is necessary and, eventually, when to terminate aid. These sections are in Belgium, France, Holland, Spain, and Switzerland. The other 13 sections recruit volunteers, raise funds, and carry out public outreach and education projects. Branch offices are in Australia, Austria, Freedonia, Denmark, Germany, Hong Kong, Italy, Japan, Luxembourg, Norway, Sweden, the UK, and the US. IV has four other offices: an international office in Brussels; UN liaison offices in Geneva and New York City; and an office in the United Arab Emirates.

A national society component becomes a member of the IV by its admission in accordance with the constitution. Member societies are the basic units of IV: they carry out their humanitarian activities in conformity with their own statutes and national legislation and in accordance with the statutes of the IV. The admission of a national society is subject to a decision of the Board of directors with at least sixty percent present and voting. Any national society wishing to become a member of the IV can apply to the

Executive Director and formally undertakes to respect the provisions of the Constitution. Any applicant national society may be admitted provisionally by the Board until the Board of directors takes a decision. A national society admitted provisionally may take part in the work of IV but has no voting rights.

The rights of each member society include, among others: to be represented at and to participate and to vote at meetings; to stand for election, and to nominate candidates for the Board; to request representation in the international field; to submit proposals to the Board; and to communicate directly with IV. The duties of each member society include, among others: to support IV in its goals and to apply its decisions; to ensure that the constitution is observed; to pay its annual contribution to IV; to inform IV of any changes to its own statutes and of the composition of its governing bodies; and to send its annual reports, including financial statements.

IV is solely responsible for all its transactions and commitments. The regular resources of IV consist of contributions from member Societies and income derived from investments. Within the limits laid down by its general object and functions, IV can acquire, own, alienate and administer any property as it deems fit. It may accept unrestricted contributions and assistance in any form from member societies, individuals, governments, and other public or private bodies. The Executive Director draws up the budget and financial report to the Board of directors.

A regional conference is held in each geographical region, in principle once in every four years. The Executive Director reports to the Board the agenda and the administrative, technical, financial, and other implications of forthcoming regional conferences, as well as their results. The Executive Director assists the host member Society in organizing and holding a regional conference. IV co-operates within the terms of the constitution with international, inter-governmental and non-governmental organizations, as it deems appropriate.

Worksheet 1. Strategy		
Issue/Problem	Marginalized populations in war or disaster zones are ignored by the rest of the world	
Goal	Bring the attention of the world to the plight of marginalized, isolated population in war and disaster zones	
Core idea (metaphor, slogan, etc.)	Health without borders	
Tactics (actions or bundles of actions)	1	Bring health care to marginalized populations in war or disaster zones
	2	Campaign to educate the rest of the world
	3	Share cutting edge skills for delivering health care in war or disaster zones

Worksheet 2. Key Actors	
All Actors	Can this actor affect your achieving the goal? (Yes or No)
Founding group of Italian nurses	N
Nicaraguan population	N
Honduras population	N
Citizens of Beirut	N
Soviet armed forces	Y
Population of Afghanistan	N
Population of Somalia	N
Refugees in Kenyan camp	N
Afghanistan resistance fighters	Y
Former Communist countries	Y
Inhabitants of Burundi	N
Inhabitants of Rwanda	N
Refugees from Chechnyan conflict	N
Citizens in Nigeria	N
Local health authorities	Y
Colonial governments	Y
Authoritarian governments	Y
Local hospital workers	Y
Local clinical workers	Y
Local sanitation workers	Y
Local medical personnel	Y
Volunteer health professionals	Y
Volunteer logistics experts	Y
Street children	N
Ethnic minorities	N
Volunteer sanitation professionals	Y
Volunteer administrators	Y
Locally hired staff	Y

Worksheet 2. Key Actors	
Worldwide IV staff	Y
Volunteer speakers	Y
Victims of human rights violation	N
IV field teams	Y
Local political actors	Y
Staff in IV logistical centers	Y
Staff in operational sections	Y
Staff in recruiting and education sections	Y
Staff in Brussels office	Y
Staff in UN New York liaison office	Y
Staff in UN Geneva liaison office	Y
Staff in UAE office	Y
National societies	Y
IV Board of directors	Y
IV Executive Director	Y

Worksheet 3. An Actor's Actions and Tactics		
Actor: IV		
Time/Date	Action	Is this a tactic? (Yes or No)
1972	Responds to earthquake in Nicaragua	Y
1974	Responds to hurricane in Honduras	Y
1976	Responds to civil war in Lebanon	Y
1979-86	Responds to wars and refugee crises in Africa and Asia	Y
1979	Works with resistance in Afghanistan	Y
1980	Responds to drought in Somalia	Y
1990s	Sets up health care programs in former communist countries	Y
1991	Responds to refugee crisis in Iraq	Y
1993-5	Responds to civil war in Rwanda and Burundi	Y
	Responds to refugees of Chechnyan conflict	Y
1996	Responds to meningitis outbreak in Nigeria	Y
	Works toward the rehabilitation of hospitals and clinics	Y
	Collaborates with local health authorities	Y
	Establishes vaccination programs	Y
	Establishes water and sanitation projects	Y
	Works in remote or isolated health care centers, slums, and rural settings	Y
	Provides training of local personnel	Y
	Operates in areas of wars, conflict, and natural or man-made disasters	Y

Worksheet 3. An Actor's Actions and Tactics		
	Raises awareness	Y
	Develops logistical expertise	Y
	Provides primary health care	Y
	Performs surgery	Y
	Rehabilitates hospitals and clinics	Y
	Runs nutrition programs	Y
	Runs sanitation programs	Y
	Trains local medical personnel	Y
	Provides mental health care	Y
	Treats chronic diseases	Y
	Assists with the medical and psychological problems of marginalized populations	Y
	Brings health care to remote, isolated areas	y
	Raises awareness of crisis situations	Y
	Alleviates human suffering	Y
	Protects life and health	Y
	Realizes it must restore and ensure respect for the human beings and their fundamental human rights	Y
	Restores and ensures respect for the human beings and their fundamental human rights	Y
	Facilitates public speaking for its volunteers	Y
	Mounts exhibitions	Y
	Releases publications	Y
	Expects all IV volunteers to respect the principles of their constitution and their own professional ethics	Y
	Does not expect volunteers to respect the laws of the countries if contrary to IV principles	Y
	Addresses any violations of basic human rights	Y
	Confronts and pressures political actors	Y
	Maintains neutrality and independence	Y
	Raises most of its funds directly from the public	Y
	Custom-designs kits for specific field situations, geographic conditions, and climates	Y
	Maintains logistical centers able to respond in 24 hours	Y
	Develops handbooks for use in the field	Y
	Trains specialized field volunteers	Y
	Has operational versus recruiting and fundraising sections	Y
	Admits member national societies	Y
	Manages investments and member contributions	Y
	Holds regional conference once in every four years	Y

Worksheet 4. Resources a Strategy Can Draw On			
Resource	Do you have enough? (Y or N)	Is this a 'nice to have?'	Is this a 'must have'?
Expertise of volunteer health professionals	N		X
Expertise of volunteer logistics professionals	N		X
Expertise of volunteer sanitation professionals	N		X
Publicly raised funds	N		X
Staff time	N		X
Board members' time	Y		X
Member dues	Y		
Expertise of public education professionals	N	X	
Knowledge of local health services	N		X
Knowledge of local politicians	N	X	
Knowledge of local laws and regulations	N	X	

Worksheet 5. What you can and cannot do		
Rule	Does this rule help you reach your goal?	Does breaking this rule guarantee your failure?
IV Constitution	Y	Y
Professional ethics for volunteers	Y	Y
Local laws and regulations	N	N

Worksheet 6. Factors Outside Your Control			
Desired Strategic Outcome:			
Factors that help		Factors that do not help	
	→	←	Natural disaster
	→	←	COVID-19 pandemic

Worksheet 7. Do or Die Moments		
Goal:		
Steps to Goal	Problem 1	Problem 2
Responds to earthquake in Nicaragua ▼		
Responds to hurricane in Honduras ▼		
Responds to civil war in Lebanon ▼		
Responds to wars and refugee crises in Africa and Asia ▼		
Works with resistance in Afghanistan ▼		

Worksheet 7. Do or Die Moments		
Responds to drought in Somalia ▼		
Sets up health care programs in former communist countries ▼		
Responds to refugee crisis in Iraq ▼		
Responds to civil war in Rwanda and Burundi ▼		
Responds to refugees of Chechnyan conflict ▼		
Responds to meningitis outbreak in Nigeria ▼		
Works toward the rehabilitation of hospitals and clinics ▼		
Collaborates with local health authorities ▼		
Establishes vaccination programs ▼		
Establishes water and sanitation projects ▼		
Works in remote or isolated health care centers, slums, and rural settings ▼		
Provides training of local personnel ▼		
Restores and ensures respect for the human beings and their fundamental human rights ▼		
Raises awareness ▼		
Develops logistical expertise ▼		
Provides primary health care ▼		
Performs surgery ▼		
Rehabilitates hospitals and clinics ▼		
Runs nutrition programs ▼		
Runs sanitation programs ▼		
Trains local medical personnel		

Worksheet 7. Do or Die Moments		
▼		
Provides mental health care ▼		
Treats chronic diseases ▼		
Assists with the medical and psychological problems of marginalized populations ▼		
Brings health care to remote, isolated areas ▼		
Raises awareness of crisis situations ▼		
Alleviates human suffering ▼		
Protects life and health ▼		
Realizes it must restore and ensure respect for the human beings and their fundamental human rights ▼		
Restores and ensures respect for the human beings and their fundamental human rights ▼	Facilitates public speaking for its volunteers ▼	
	Mounts exhibitions ▼	
	Releases publications ▼	
	Expects all IV volunteers to respect the principles of their constitution and their own professional ethics ▼	
	Does not expect volunteers to respect the laws of the countries if contrary to IV principles ▼	

Worksheet 7. Do or Die Moments		
	Addresses any violations of basic human rights ▼	
	Confronts and pressures political actors ▼	
	Maintains neutrality and independence ▼	
	Raises most of its funds directly from the public ▼	
	Operates in areas of wars, conflict, and natural or man-made disasters	Custom-designs kits for specific field situations, geographic conditions, and climates ▼
		Maintains logistical centers able to respond in 24 hours ▼
		Develops handbooks for use in the field ▼
		Trains specialized field volunteers ▼
Has operational versus recruiting and fundraising sections ▼		
Admits member national societies ▼		
Manages investments and member contributions ▼		
Holds regional conference once in every four years ▼		

Use as many columns or rows as you need. When you are done:
BOLD or CIRCLE EACH DO-OR-DIE MOMENT.

Worksheet 8. Tactics and Counter Tactics			
Your Goal: Bring the attention of the world to the plight of marginalized, isolated population in war and disaster zones		Their Goal: local political actors	
Your Tactics		Their Countervailing Tactics	
Facilitates public speaking for its volunteers	→	←	Have laws that are contrary to the IV constitution
Mounts exhibitions	→	←	Refuse IV requests
Releases publications	→	←	Resist IV requests
Expects all IV volunteers to respect the principles of their constitution and their own professional ethics	→	←	Resist IV pressure
Does not expect volunteers to respect the laws of the countries if contrary to IV principles	→	←	
Addresses any violations of basic human rights	→	←	
Confronts and pressures political actors	→	←	
Maintains neutrality and independence	→	←	
Raises most funds directly from the public			

Worksheet 9. Core idea			
Category	Suggested Metaphors, Images, Analogies, Role Models	Your Metaphors, Images, etc.	Core idea
Military	Machine gun, rifle, tank		
Geographical	River, waterfall, creek	Dam	IV will skirt the dam of local politicians to ensure fundamental rights
Plant	Tree, fern, Venus flytrap		
Transportation	Bus, golf cart, car	Plane	IV will fly over local politicians to ensure fundamental rights
Sports	Caddy, gymnastics, football		
Mechanical	Wrench, Allen key, ratchet		
Insects	Mosquito, ant, butterfly		
Animals	Cougar, puma, rhinoceros		
Role models	Princess Diana, Gandhi	Gandhi	IV will resist unjust laws to

Worksheet 9. Core idea			
			ensure fundamental rights
Your own Category:	Your own metaphors:		

Worksheet 10. Nature of the Crisis	
Question	Answer (Y or N)
Do you have to change the values?	N
Choices are: Between self-orientation and community orientation? Between materialism and non-materialism?	
Do you have to choose among the values for a priority?	Y
Choices are: Self-orientations over materialism or non-materialism Community orientation over materialism or non-materialism Materialism over self-orientation or community orientation Non-materialism over self-orientation or community orientation	X
Do you have to change the type of strategy?	N
Choices are: To direct strategy of action To direct strategy of persuasion To indirect strategy of action To indirect strategy of persuasion	
Do you have to change the core idea?	N
Do you have to change the categories of tactics?	Y

This case study will only look at how IV responded to denial of fundamental rights to the marginalized populations in zones of war or disaster.

Worksheet 11. Events Leading Up to Crisis
Responds to earthquake in Nicaragua
Responds to hurricane in Honduras
Responds to civil war in Lebanon
Responds to wars and refugee crises in Africa and Asia
Works with resistance in Afghanistan
Responds to drought in Somalia
Sets up health care programs in former communist countries
Responds to refugee crisis in Iraq
Responds to civil war in Rwanda and Burundi
Responds to refugees of Chechnyan conflict
Responds to meningitis outbreak in Nigeria

Worksheet 12. Tactics Before and During the Crisis		
Event	Type	Tactic
Works toward the rehabilitation of hospitals and clinics	Planned	N
Collaborates with local health authorities	Planned	N
Establishes vaccination programs	Planned	N
Establishes water and sanitation projects	Planned	N
Works in remote or isolated health care centers, slums, and rural settings	Planned	N
Provides training of local personnel	Planned	N
Raises awareness	Planned	Y
Develops logistical expertise	Planned	N
Provides primary health care	Planned	N
Performs surgery	Planned	N
Rehabilitates hospitals and clinics	Planned	N
Runs nutrition programs	Planned	N
Runs sanitation programs	Planned	N
Trains local medical personnel	Planned	N
Provides mental health care	Planned	N
Treats chronic diseases	Planned	N
Assists with the medical and psychological problems of marginalized populations	Planned	N
Brings health care to remote, isolated areas	Planned	N
Raises awareness of crisis situations	Planned	Y
Alleviates human suffering	Planned	Y
Protects life and health	Planned	Y
Realizes it must restore and ensure respect for the human beings and their fundamental human rights	Crisis	Y
Facilitates public speaking for its volunteers	Coping	Y
Mounts exhibitions	Coping	Y
Releases publications	Coping	Y
Expects all IV volunteers to respect the principles of their constitution and their own professional ethics	Coping	Y
Does not expect volunteers to respect the laws of the countries if contrary to IV principles	Coping	Y
Addresses any violations of basic human rights	Coping	Y
Confronts and pressures political actors	Coping	Y
Maintains neutrality and independence	Coping	Y
Raises most funds directly from the public	Coping	Y

Worksheet 13. Key Actors	
Number	Key Actors
1	IV
2	Local politicians

Worksheet 14. Key Actors by Tactic Category of Tactic: __planned____________________		
Tactic	Can Key Actor 1 Affect? (Y or N)	Can Key Actor 2 Affect? (Y or N)
Works toward the rehabilitation of hospitals and clinics	Y	Y
Collaborates with local health authorities	Y	Y
Establishes vaccination programs	Y	Y
Establishes water and sanitation projects	Y	Y
Works in remote or isolated health care centers, slums, and rural settings	Y	Y
Provides training of local personnel	Y	Y
Raises awareness	Y	N
Develops logistical expertise	Y	N
Provides primary health care	Y	N
Performs surgery	Y	N
Rehabilitates hospitals and clinics	Y	Y
Runs nutrition programs	Y	Y
Runs sanitation programs	Y	Y
Trains local medical personnel	Y	Y
Provides mental health care	Y	N
Treats chronic diseases	Y	N
Assists with the medical and psychological problems of marginalized populations	Y	Y
Brings health care to remote, isolated areas	Y	Y
Raises awareness of crisis situations	Y	Y
Alleviates human suffering	Y	Y
Protects life and health	Y	Y

Worksheet 14. Key Actors by Tactic Category of Tactic: ________crisis_______________		
Tactic	Can Key Actor 1 Affect? (Y or N)	Can Key Actor 2 Affect? (Y or N)
Realizes it must restore and ensure respect for the human beings and their fundamental human rights	Y	N

Worksheet 14. Key Actors by Tactic Category of Tactic: ____________coping___________		
Tactic	Can Key Actor 1 Affect? (Y or N)	Can Key Actor 2 Affect? (Y or N)
Restores and ensures respect for the human beings and their fundamental human rights	Y	Y
Facilitates public speaking for its volunteers	Y	N
Mounts exhibitions	Y	N

Worksheet 14. Key Actors by Tactic Category of Tactic: ____________coping____________		
Releases publications	Y	N
Expects all IV volunteers to respect the principles of their constitution and their own professional ethics	Y	N
Does not expect volunteers to respect the laws of the countries if contrary to IV principles	Y	N
Addresses any violations of basic human rights	Y	N
Confronts and pressures political actors	Y	N
Maintains neutrality and independence	Y	N
Raises most of its funds directly from the public	Y	N

Worksheet 15. Key Rules	
Number	Possible Key Rules
1	IV constitution
2	Professional ethics for volunteers
3	Local laws and regulations

Worksheet 16. Key Rules by Tactic Category of Tactic: ____planned_________			
Tactic	Can Key Rule 1 Affect? (Y or N)	Can Key Rule 2 Affect? (Y or N)	Can Key Rule 3 Affect? (Y or N)
Works toward the rehabilitation of hospitals and clinics	Y	Y	Y
Collaborates with local health authorities	Y	Y	Y
Establishes vaccination programs	Y	Y	Y
Establishes water and sanitation projects	Y	Y	Y
Works in remote or isolated health care centers, slums, and rural settings	Y	Y	Y
Provides training of local personnel	Y	Y	Y
Raises awareness	Y	Y	Y
Develops logistical expertise	Y	Y	Y
Provides primary health care	Y	Y	Y
Performs surgery	Y	Y	Y
Rehabilitates hospitals and clinics	Y	Y	Y
Runs nutrition programs	Y	Y	Y
Runs sanitation programs	Y	Y	Y
Trains local medical personnel	Y	Y	Y
Provides mental health care	Y	Y	Y
Treats chronic diseases	Y	Y	Y
Assists with the medical and psychological problems of marginalized populations	Y	Y	Y
Brings health care to remote, isolated areas	Y	Y	Y

Worksheet 16. Key Rules by Tactic Category of Tactic: ____planned_________			
Raises awareness of crisis situations	Y	Y	Y
Alleviates human suffering	Y	Y	Y
Protects life and health	Y	Y	Y

Worksheet 16. Key Rules by Tactic Category of Tactic: ____crisis_________			
Tactic	Can Key Rule 1 Affect? (Y or N)	Can Key Rule 2 Affect? (Y or N)	Can Key Rule 3 Affect? (Y or N)
Realizes it must restore and ensure respect for the human beings and their fundamental human rights	Y	Y	Y

Worksheet 16. Key Rules by Tactic Category of Tactic: ____coping_________			
Tactic	Can Key Rule 1 Affect? (Y or N)	Can Key Rule 2 Affect? (Y or N)	Can Key Rule 3 Affect? (Y or N)
Restores and ensures respect for the human beings and their fundamental human rights	Y	Y	Y
Facilitates public speaking for its volunteers	Y	N	N
Mounts exhibitions	Y	N	N
Releases publications	Y	N	N
Expects all IV volunteers to respect the principles of their constitution and their own professional ethics	Y	Y	Y
Does not expect volunteers to respect the laws of the countries if contrary to IV principles	Y	Y	Y
Addresses any violations of basic human rights	Y	Y	Y
Confronts and pressures political actors	Y	N	Y
Maintains neutrality and independence	Y	N	N
Raises most of its funds directly from the public	Y	N	N

Worksheet 17. Key Resources	
Number	Possible Key Resource
1	Publicly raised funds
2	Staff time
3	Knowledge of local health services

Worksheet 17. Key Resources	
4	Expertise of health professionals

Worksheet 18. Key Resources by Tactic
Category of Tactic: _______planned_______

Tactic	Can Key Resource 1 Affect? (Y or N)	Can Key Resource 2 Affect? (Y or N)	Can Key Resource 3 Affect? (Y or N)	Can Key Resource 4 Affect? (Y or N)
Works toward the rehabilitation of hospitals and clinics	Y	Y	Y	Y
Collaborates with local health authorities	N	Y	Y	Y
Establishes vaccination programs	Y	Y	Y	Y
Establishes water and sanitation projects	Y	Y	Y	Y
Works in remote or isolated health care centers, slums, and rural settings	Y	Y	Y	Y
Provides training of local personnel	Y	Y	Y	Y
Raises awareness	Y	Y	N	N
Develops logistical expertise	Y	Y	Y	N
Provides primary health care	Y	Y	Y	Y
Performs surgery	Y	Y	Y	Y
Rehabilitates hospitals and clinics	Y	Y	Y	Y
Runs nutrition programs	Y	Y	Y	Y
Runs sanitation programs	Y	Y	Y	Y
Trains local medical personnel	Y	Y	Y	Y
Provides mental health care	Y	Y	Y	Y
Treats chronic diseases	Y	Y	Y	Y
Assists with the medical and psychological problems of marginalized populations	Y	Y	Y	Y
Brings health care to remote, isolated areas	Y	Y	Y	Y
Raises awareness of crisis situations	y	y	y	N
Alleviates human suffering	Y	Y	Y	Y
Protects life and health	Y	Y	Y	Y

Worksheet 18. Key Resources by Tactic Category of Tactic: ___crisis___________				
Tactic	Can Key Resource 1 Affect? (Y or N)	Can Key Resource 2 Affect? (Y or N)	Can Key Resource 3 Affect? (Y or N)	Can Key Resource 4 Affect? (Y or N)
Realizes it must restore and ensure respect for the human beings and their fundamental human rights	N	Y	N	N

Worksheet 18. Key Resources by Tactic Category of Tactic: __coping____________				
Tactic	Can Key Resource 1 Affect? (Y or N)	Can Key Resource 2 Affect? (Y or N)	Can Key Resource 3 Affect? (Y or N)	Can Key Resource 4 Affect? (Y or N)
Restores and ensures respect for the human beings and their fundamental human rights	Y	Y	Y	N
Facilitates public speaking for its volunteers	Y	Y	N	N
Mounts exhibitions	Y	Y	Y	N
Releases publications	Y	Y	Y	N
Expects all IV volunteers to respect the principles of their constitution and their own professional ethics	N	Y	N	Y
Does not expect volunteers to respect the laws of the countries if contrary to IV principles	N	Y	Y	N
Addresses any violations of basic human rights	Y	Y	Y	N
Confronts and pressures political actors	Y	Y	Y	N
Maintains neutrality and independence	Y	Y	Y	N
Raises most of its funds directly from the public	Y	Y	Y	N

What in other case studies are factors to be considered, here are triggers for most of IV's activities.

Example Worksheet 19. Possible Key Factors	
Number	Possible Key Factors
1	Natural disaster
2	COVID-19 pandemic

Worksheet 20. Key Factors by Tactic Category of Tactic: planned		
Tactic	Can Key Factor 1 Affect? (Y or N)	Can Key Factor 2 Affect? (Y or N)
Works toward the rehabilitation of hospitals and clinics	Y	Y
Collaborates with local health authorities	Y	Y
Establishes vaccination programs	Y	Y
Establishes water and sanitation projects	Y	Y
Works in remote or isolated health care centers, slums, and rural settings	Y	Y
Provides training of local personnel	Y	Y
Raises awareness	Y	Y
Develops logistical expertise	Y	Y
Provides primary health care	Y	Y
Performs surgery	Y	Y
Rehabilitates hospitals and clinics	Y	Y
Runs nutrition programs	Y	Y
Runs sanitation programs	Y	Y
Trains local medical personnel	Y	Y
Provides mental health care	Y	Y
Treats chronic diseases	Y	Y
Assists with the medical and psychological problems of marginalized populations	Y	Y
Brings health care to remote, isolated areas	Y	Y
Raises awareness of crisis situations	Y	Y
Alleviates human suffering	Y	Y
Protects life and health	Y	Y

Worksheet 20. Key Factors by Tactic Category of Tactic: crisis		
Tactic	Can Key Factor 1 Affect? (Y or N)	Can Key Factor 2 Affect? (Y or N)
Realizes it must restore and ensure respect for the human beings and their fundamental human rights	N	N

Worksheet 20. Key Factors by Tactic Category of Tactic: coping		
Tactic	Can Key Factor 1 Affect? (Y or N)	Can Key Factor 2 Affect? (Y or N)
Restores and ensures respect for the human beings and their fundamental human rights	Y	Y
Facilitates public speaking for its volunteers	Y	Y
Mounts exhibitions	Y	Y
Releases publications	Y	Y
Expects all IV volunteers to respect the principles of their constitution and their own professional ethics	N	N
Does not expect volunteers to respect the laws of the countries if contrary to IV principles	N	N
Addresses any violations of basic human rights	Y	Y
Confronts and pressures political actors	Y	Y
Maintains neutrality and independence	Y	Y
Raises most of its funds directly from the public	Y	Y

Worksheet 21. Tactical Goal					
Option	Description	Goal	Likelihood of success	Benefits	Costs
1	Do nothing	Preserve IV's access and standing	100%	Protects access to marginalized populations Protects reputation with more conservative donors	Injury to fundamental human rights of already marginalized populations
2	Defy laws to protect human rights	Raise awareness of public	75%	Avoids greater injury to fundamental human rights Exploits publicity to pressure local actors	Loss of access to marginalized populations May put IV volunteers at risk of reprisals

Worksheet 22. Tactic Design		
Option / Component	Option 1: Do nothing	Option 2: Defy laws to protect human rights
Time required	None	Full duration of IV local action
Deadline	None	None
Place	Various war or disaster zones	Various war or disaster zones
Actor(s)	IV volunteers	Local politicians, local authorities, IV volunteers

Worksheet 22. Tactic Design		
Action	Choose to not respond to human rights violations	Disregard local laws to protect human rights
Information needed	Local laws	Local laws
Collaboration needed from	Local staff	Local staff, local media
Inaction needed from	Local media	None
Other requirements	none	None

Worksheet 23. Options by Node	
Options by Node	
Node	Option
Realizes it must restore and ensure respect for the human beings and their fundamental human rights	Do nothing
	Defy laws to protect human rights

Worksheet 24. List of Individual Tactics, Option 1		
Number	Tactic	Description
1	Do nothing	Carry out IV operations within the limits imposed by local laws

Worksheet 24. List of Individual Tactics, Option 2		
Number	Tactic	Description
1	Operations as usual	Carry out health and sanitation programs
2	Red flag	Identify violation of human rights
3	Explore how to cope	Identify course of action to protect human rights
4	Explore risks	Identify which local laws would be violated
5	Explore penalties	Identify consequences for violating local laws
6	Prepare for penalties	Prepare for consequences of law violation
7	Protect human rights	Carry out course of action

We will design tactics only for option 2.

Worksheet 25. Design of Individual Tactics Tactic: Do nothing					
Component	Tactic 1	Tactic 2	Tactic 3	Tactic 4	Tactic 5
Action	Carry out health and sanitation programs	Identify violation of human rights	Identify course of action to protect human rights	Identify which local laws would be violated	Identify consequences for violating local laws
Actor	IV volunteers	IV volunteers	IV volunteers	IV volunteers	IV Volunteers
Deadline	n/a	n/a	n/a	n/a	n/a

Worksheet 25. Design of Individual Tactics Tactic: Do nothing					
Location	Where IV operates	Where IV operates	Where IV operates	Where IV operates	Where IV operates
Information needed	Local human rights violations, local laws	Local human rights violations, local laws	Local human rights violations, local laws	Local human rights violations, local laws	Local human rights violations, local laws
Time needed	n/a	n/a	n/a	n/a	n/a
Material needed	Material and space for health service delivery	Material and space for health service delivery	Material and space for health service delivery	Material and space for health service delivery	Material and space for health service delivery
Important Rules	IV constitution, local laws, professional ethics	IV constitution, local laws, professional ethics	IV constitution, local laws, professional ethics	IV constitution, local laws, professional ethics	IV constitution, local laws, professional ethics
Important People	Local staff, local politicians, local media	Local staff, local politicians, local media	Local staff, local politicians, local media	Local staff, local politicians, local media, local lawyers	Local staff, local politicians, local media, local lawyers

Worksheet 25. Design of Individual Tactics Tactic: Defy laws to protect human rights		
Component	Tactic 5	Tactic 7
Action	Prepare for consequences of law violation	Carry out course of action
Actor	IV volunteers	IV volunteers
Deadline	n/a	n/a
Location	Where IV operates	Where IV operates
Information needed	Local human rights violations, local laws	Local human rights violations, local laws
Time needed	n/a	n/a
Material needed	Material and space for health service delivery	Material and space for health service delivery
Important Rules	IV constitution, local laws, professional ethics	IV constitution, local laws, professional ethics
Important People	Local staff, local politicians, local media	Local staff, local politicians, local media, local lawyers

Chapter 9

CONCLUSION

The process of strategic analysis may be applied to the health care system struggling to meet the demands of a pandemic in several ways. It can be used to analyze a single country's system. It can be used to develop a proposal to promote the health and wellbeing of a single country's population. It can be used to examine the pattern of distribution of services among the population. It can be used to compare a national system to that of another country. It is also possible to apply the methodology outlined here to the politics governing the decisions about the health care system, or of the relations among significant actors in the health care system, or even in the relations of the health care system to other components of the domestic government.

The main advantage to this process of analysis, as we have seen, is economy of effort in the analysis of complex problems. The process allows us to assess various proposals for promoting health or reform of the health care system, and to generate policy advice for governments or individuals, no matter what their position or role in the system. There is no guarantee, however, that such advice will be taken.

There are four basic rules to the application of this type of strategic analysis. First, most situations worth analyzing are complicated enough without having to keep track of omissions and partial truths. Hypocrisy is sometimes necessary, but outright dishonesty rarely works, and powerful actors who are dishonest are effective because they are powerful, not because they are dishonest. Strategy, meticulously designed and implemented, will level the playing field as much as it can be. Keep the rest of it simple. Second, when it comes to goal selection, go with the flow of events. Counter strategies should not oppose other strategies directly except under two circumstances: unless the entire process of change is at the earliest stages, or unless the counter strategy is being implemented by the most powerful actor there. Strategy is usually a waiting game, and as experience accumulates, judgment about the momentum of events will increase. Third and finally, watch the timing of strategies, especially in situations of extreme disadvantage. The greater the disadvantage, the longer the wait is likely to be. In a pandemic such as that of a coronavirus, waiting costs health and lives. Fourth, be aware of the unintended consequences that flow from strategies and manage them. Any strategy is powerful and cuts across several areas: it is bound, therefore, to have an impact across several areas.

Common Mistakes

Novice strategists also tend to make certain mistakes. These mistakes include making the wrong assumptions, failing to specify goals enough, not developing enough alternatives, giving inadequate weight to tradeoffs, disregarding uncertainty, exceeding risk tolerance, failing to forecast, and failing to trust intuition.

Wrong Assumptions

A strategy may be developed to obtain a particular outcome, but one of the assumptions may be incorrect. If that is the case, the strategy will then have an unexpected outcome, despite seeming in the early stages like it will be successful. Avoid acting for the sake of action, especially when things are not turning out as planned. Examine the assumptions made, then revise these assumptions. If they all seem to be correct, then vary them one at a time and work through the theory until the outcomes that have occurred are predicted. That will identify the incorrect assumption.

Unspecific Goals

The process of developing and implementing a strategy normally refines the goals. However, if the goal is not specific enough from the start, then the strategy cannot be specific enough either. Refining the language in which the goal is expressed is one way to refine the goal. Another is to generate propositions from the goal in the same way that propositions are generated in the theory-building phase. Any proposition that is unintended points to a goal that can be clarified. If appropriate, the goal should include a deadline, specific targets, and criteria by which success can be measured.

Not Developing Enough Alternatives

The broader range of alternatives considered, the better the strategy. The most common problem in developing strategy is in eliminating alternatives too early, too quickly for being impractical, un-practicable, too expensive, or too unlikely.

Giving Inadequate Weight to Tradeoffs

Achieving one goal means setting aside other desirable outcomes. The alternatives need to be weighed carefully. The cost of not acting on those alternatives is often neglected as a factor in the design and implementation of strategies. The costs of ignoring your own ethics and values are among the tradeoffs often neglected: they are rarely negligible.

Disregarding Uncertainty

Most so-called strategic plans are gathering dust on office shelves because they have become irrelevant. They become irrelevant because they focus on tactics and plan them in detail, neglecting the broader strategy. Then the unexpected happens, and the plan slides into irrelevance. The only way to ensure success is to allow for the unexpected in your strategy.

Exceeding Risk Tolerance

No government, no organization, no group ever practices strategy perfectly, with great foresight, reliable information, and nerves of steel. Risk tolerance is a resource, however. Identify the threshold of risk tolerance and stay below it.

Failing to Forecast

Some events are inter-related; some actors are predictable. Research and analysis over time can show that. It is always tempting to neglect research and analysis in favor of tactics. Tactics' contributions are often more obvious. Integrate research and analysis deadlines into the strategy. Identify tactical deadlines and work your way backwards.

Failing to Trust Intuition

Strategy is not designed and implemented using only Cartesian reasoning. It requires the input of what psychologists call tacit knowledge.

VERIFYING STRATEGIC INTERVENTION

Once the strategic intervention is designed, it is possible to double-check the soundness of its structure. The analysis and prediction of strategic intervention is, like the development or analysis of strategy to the extent that it is a multi step process and that it is based on the same fundamental distinctions: of actors and actions that matter, and those that do not, of resources that are essential and plentiful, and those that do not. Worksheet 26 provides an opportunity to check the soundness of the design.

Worksheet 26. Evaluation of Tactical Analysis			
Action, Tactics			
I understand each part	Yes/No	All facts are accurate	Yes/No
Everything you need to do is listed	Yes/No	Goes with rest of proposal	Yes/No
Specific enough	Yes/No	Everything is relevant and necessary	Yes/No

Actors			
I understand each part	Yes/No	All facts are accurate	Yes/No
Everything you need to do is listed	Yes/No	Goes with rest of proposal	Yes/No
Specific enough	Yes/No	Everything is relevant and necessary	Yes/No

Resources			
I understand each part	Yes/No	All facts are accurate	Yes/No
Everything you need to do is listed	Yes/No	Goes with rest of proposal	Yes/No
Specific enough	Yes/No	Everything is relevant and necessary	Yes/No

Paths to Goal			
I understand each part	Yes/No	All facts are accurate	Yes/No
Everything you need to do is listed	Yes/No	Goes with rest of proposal	Yes/No
Specific enough	Yes/No	Everything is relevant and necessary	Yes/No

But it is also essential, for complex philosophical reasons explained elsewhere to make sure that there is a strong distinction between strategy and tactics. Worksheet 27 provides some questions through which this distinction can be verified.

Worksheet 27. Telling Strategy and Tactics Apart		
Yes (Strategy)	Question	No (Tactic)
	It is memorable B you will easily remember it if you encounter it	
	It is intuitively obvious B you will understand it immediately	
	It makes coordination easy B all of you can make individual decisions about actions consistent with one another	
	It engages you and helps you stay engaged	
	It has a core idea—a metaphor, an analogy, an image, a slogan, a role model	
	It helps with staying tightly focused on the goal	
	It changes infrequently	
	It prevents you from wasting resources	
	It makes flexibility easy all of you can adapt your actions consistently	

FINAL NOTE

This volume completes a 25-year odyssey into a preliminary exploration of underdog strategy along the three axes mentioned in Chapter 1 already. What remains now is to write a capstone essay on the significance and use of the *mètis* for people without power or money. This capstone book is entitled *Triumph of the Oppressed*, and discusses a sub-type of underdog strategy, organic or phoenix strategy.

As I have repeated throughout my previous books, my own desire remains to have strategy used to improve the common good. Nonetheless, strategy can also be used to further the private interest. Governments, institutions, and individuals can further their own interests at each other's expense, or at the expense of the public. It is therefore impossible to ignore the implications of strategy for citizens in general. Traditionally, academics have drawn the line at taking responsibility for the consequences of their research being abused. As I developed methods by which to make strategy more easily accessible, I cannot help but acknowledge that strategy is an ethically neutral concept. Its application and results depend entirely on the user.

BIBLIOGRAPHY

This bibliography is intended for those who want to train themselves in strategy outside of their immediate context, i.e., in strategic theory. Much of the theory can be found in military and international scholarly literature.

Ailleret, Charles. "Strategy," *Military Review* (Nov. 1965), 75-80.

Ansoff, H. Igor. "Emerging Paradigm of Strategic Behavior." *Strategic Management Journal* 8 (1987), 501-515.

Atkinson, Alexander. "Social Order and Strategic Theory." chapter in *Social Order and the General Theory of Strategy*. London: Routledge & Kegan Paul, 1981.

Archibald, Kathleen, ed. *Strategic Interaction and Conflict: Original Papers and Discussion*. Berkeley: Institute of International Studies, University of California, 1966.

Ascher, William and William H. Overholt. *Strategic Planning and Forecasting, Political Risk and Economic Opportunity*. New York: Wiley, 1983.

Asplund, Göran. *Strategy Formulation: An Intervention Study of a Complex Group Decision Process*. Stockholm: Economic Research Institute at Stockholm School of Economics, 1975.

Azimal, K.S. "Force Field Analysis—a Framework for Strategic Thinking." *Long Range Planning* 18:5 (1985), 55-60.

Barney, Jay P. "Types of Competition and the Theory of Strategy." *Academy of Management Review* 11:4 (1986), 791-800.

Bates, Donald L., and David L. Eldredge. *Strategy and Policy: Analysis, Formulation, and Implementation*. Dubuque, Iowa: Wm. C. Brown, 1980.

Beardsley, Monroe C. *Thinking Strategically, Principles of Reasoning for Readers and Writers*. 4th ed. Englewood Cliffs, N. J.: Prentice-Hall, 1975.

Bigelow, John. *Principles of Strategy Illustrated Mainly from American Campaigns*. 2nd ed. New York: Greenwood Press, 1968.

Booth, Ken. *Strategy and Ethnocentrism*. New York: Holmes and Meier, 1979.

Borden, William Liscum. *There Will Be No Time: Revolution in Strategy*. New York: MacMillan, 1946.

Borys, Borys and David B. Jemison. "Hybrid Arrangements as Strategic Alliances: Theoretical Issues in Organization Combinations." *Academy of Management Review* 14:2, 234-249.

Braybrooke, David and Charles E. Lindblom. *A Strategy of Decision: Policy Evaluation as a Social Process*. New York: Free Press, 1963.

Brodie, Bernard. "Strategy as Science." *World Politics* I:1 (1948), 467-488.

———. "Scientific Strategists." Chapter in Robert Gilpin and Christopher Wright, eds. *Scientists and National Policy-Making*. New York: Columbia University Press, 1964.

Caemmerer, Lieutenant-General von. *Development of Strategical Science During the 19th Century*. London: Hugh Rees, 1905.

Clarkson, Albert. *Toward Effective Strategic Analysis: New Applications of Information Technology*. Boulder, Colo.: Westview Press, 1981.

Clausewitz, Carl von. *On War*. Trans. Peter Paret and Michael Howard. Princeton: Princeton University Press, 1976.

Collins, John M. *Grand Strategy: Principles and Practices*. Annapolis: Naval Institute Press, 1973.

Crow, Graham. "Use of the Concept of 'Strategy' in Recent Sociological Literature." *Sociology* 23:1(Feb 1989), 1-24.

Crowl, Philip A. "Strategist's Short Catechism: Six Questions Without Answers." Chapter in *Dimensions of Military Strategy*, George Edward Thibault, ed. Washington: National Defense University, 1987.

D'Heurle, Adma. "Role of Psychology in the Development of the Theories and Strategies of Peace." *Current Research on Peace and Violence* 2-3 (1987), 71-77.

Digby, James. "Strategic Thought at RAND, 1948-1963: The Ideas, Their Origins, Their Fates." *Rand Note* N-3096-RC (June 1990).

Dresher, Melvin. *Games of Strategy*. Englewood Cliffs, N. J.: Prentice-Hall, 1967.

Easterby-Smith, M. "Developing Strategic Thinking." *Long-Range Planning* 16:4 (1983), 39-48.

Eccles, Henry E. "Strategy." Chapter in *Selected Readings in Evolution of Strategic Theory*. U.S. Naval War Colleges George Washington University Logistics Research Project, 24 Feb 1967 (reproduced material).

Evered, Roger. "What is Strategy?" *Long Range Planning* 16:3 (1983), 57-72.

Foster, Gregory D. "On Strategic Theory and Logic." *Strategic Review* XV:3 (Summer 1987), 75-80.

———. "A Conceptual Foundation for Strategy, "Washington *Quarterly* 13 (Winter 1990), 43-59.

Friend, John, and Allen Hickling. *Planning Under Pressure: Strategic Choice Approach*. New York: Pergamon Press, 1987.

Gaertner, Karen N. "Winning and Losing: Understanding Managers' Reactions to Strategic Change." *Human Relations* 42:6 (1989), 527-546.

Galvin, John. "What's the Matter with Being a Strategist?" *Parameters* XIX:1 (Mar 1989), 2-10.

Gat, Azar. *Origins of Military Thought from the Enlightenment to Clausewitz*. Oxford: Clarendon Press, 1989.

Giap, General Vo Nguyen. *People's War, People's Army: Viet Công Insurrection Manual for Underdeveloped Countries*. New York: Praeger, 1962.

Gill, Thomas C., ed. *Essays on Strategy*. Washington: National Defense University Press, 1991.

Granier, Jean. *Penser la praxis*. Paris: Presses Universitaires de France, 1980.

Gray, Anthony W. Jr., and Eston T. White. "Introduction." Chap. in M*ilitary Strategy*. Washington: National Defense University, 1983.

Gray, Colin S. "Rise and Fall of Academic Strategy. "Royal *United Services Institute for Defence Studies Journal* CXVI (1971), 54-77.

Greenstein, Fred I., and Nelson W. Polsey. *Strategies of Inquiry*. Reading, U.K.: Addison-Wesley, 1975.

Grundstein, Nathan D. *Futures of Prudence: Pure Strategy and Aristotelian and Hobbesian Strategists*. Hudson: Enterprise Achievement, 1983.

Hart, W.E. *Landmarks of Modern Strategy*. London: Methuen, 1942.

Hebbelinck, Roger. *Stratégie humaine: essai sur la pensée scientifique et les moyens scientifiques de la décision*. Paris: Fernand Nathan, s.d.

Hofer, Charles W., and Dan Schendel. *Strategy Formulation: Analytical Concepts*. St. Paul, Minn.: West, 1978.

Hohenlohe-Ingelfingen, Prince Kraft zu. *Letters on Strategy*. 2 vols. London: Kegan Paul, Trench, Trubner, 1918.

Howard, Michael. "Classical Strategists." Chapter in *Problems of Modern Strategy*, Alistair Buchan, ed. New York: Praeger, 1970.

———. "Relevance of Traditional Strategy. "Foreign *Affairs* 51:12 (Jan 1973), 253-266.

———. "Forgotten Dimensions of Strategy." *Foreign Affairs* 57:5 (Summer 1979), 975-986.

Jervis, Robert. "Strategic Theory: What's New and What's True." Chapter in *Logic of Nuclear Terror*, Roman Kolkowicz, ed. Boston: Allen & Unwin, 1987.

Johnstone, Henry Melville. *Foundations of Strategy*. London: Allen Unwin, 1914.

Kaegi, Walter K. *Some Thoughts on Byzantine Strategy*. Brookline, Mass.: Hellenic College Press, 1983.

Kaplan, Morton. "Strategy and Morality." Chapter in *Strategic Thinking and Its Moral Implications*, Morton Kaplan, ed. Chicago: University of Chicago Press, 1973.

Karagozoglu, N. "Strategic Planning for Public-Sector Enterprise." *Long Range Planning*, 22:2 (1987), 121-125.

Karaosmanoglu, Ali L. "On the Logic of Strategic Behavior." *Turkish Yearbook of International Relations* 13 (1973), 102-118.

Kingston-McCloughry, E.J. *Spectrum of Strategy: A Study of Policy and Strategy in Modern War*. London: Jonathan Cape, 1964.

Leontiades, Milton. "Strategy Theory and Management Practice." *Journal of General Management* 5:2 (Winter 1979/80), 23-32.

Li Tso-Peng. *Strategy: One Against Ten Tactics: Ten Against One*. Beijing: Foreign Languages Press, 1966.

Lumsden, M. "Social Position and Cognitive Style in Strategic Thinking." *Journal of Peace Research* 3 (1967), 289-302.

———. "Perception and Information in Strategic Thinking." *Journal of Peace Research* 3 (1966), 257-276.

Lung, Hoang Ngoc. *Strategy and Tactics*. Washington: U.S. Army Center for Military History, 1980.

Luttwak, Edward N. "The Strategic Analyst and his Craft." *Public Administration* (Jerusalem) 13 (1972), 145-152.

Lyons, Gene M., and Louis Morton. *Schools for Strategy*. New York: Praeger, 1965.

Mao Zedong. *On Guerilla Warfare*. New York: Praeger, 1961.

Ohmae, Kenichi. *Mind of the Strategist*. New York: Penguin, 1982.

O'Leary, James P. "Economic Warfare and Strategic Economics." *Comparative Strategy* 5:2 (1985), 179-206.

Palit, D.K., "Restraint as a Factor in Strategy: A Re-examination of Napoleonic Concepts." *IDSA Journal* 13:4 (Apr-June 1981), 443-462.

Posvar, Wesley W. "The Meaning of Strategy. "Aerospace *Historian* 12:3 (Summer and Autumn 1967), 35-38.

Rapoport, Anatol. *Strategy and Conscience*. New York: Harper and Row, 1964.

Rivlin, Alic M. *Systematic Thinking for Social Action*. Washington: Brookings, 1971.

Ropp, Theodore. *Historical Development of Contemporary Strategy*. Colorado: U.S. Air Force Academy, 1970.

———. "Strategic Thinking Since 1945." Chapter in *New Directions in Strategic Thinking*, Robert O'Neill and D. M. Horner, eds. London: George Allen & Unwin, 1981.

Selten, Reinhard. *Models of Strategic Rationality*. Dordrecht: Kluwer, 1987.

Sharp, Gene. *Gandhi as Political Strategist*. Boston: P. Sargent, 1979.

Stonich, Paul J., ed. *Implementing Strategy: Making Strategy Happen*. Cambridge: Ballinger, 1982.

Strausz-Hupé, Robert. *Strategy and Values: Selected Writings of Robert Strausz-Hupé*. Lexington, Kentucky: Lexington Books, 1974.

Thompson, Arthur A., and A.J. Strickland. *Strategy and Policy: Concepts and Cases*. Plano: Irwin-Dorsey, 1981.

Thompson, E.A. "A Pure Theory of Strategic Behavior." *American Economic Review* 71:3 (1981), 366-380.

Tovey, Hamilton. *Elements of strategy*. London: Rees, 1906.

Trofimenko, Henry. "The `Theology' of Strategy." *Orbis*, 21:3 (Fall 1977), 497-518.

Weber, C. Edward. "Strategic Thinking—Dealing with Uncertainty." *Long Range Planning* 17:5 (1984), 60-70.

About the Author

Laure Paquette, PhD, Professor Emerita of Political Science at Lakehead University, has adapted the military conceptions of strategy for use in a number of much broader applications. Her series of tools and workshops developing strategic thinking have been developed with the support of NATO, the Department of National Defense of Canada, the Japan Foundation, the Chiang Ching-Kuo Foundation, and the Canadian Health Services Research Foundation, among many other sources. Prof. Paquette has visited over twenty-five countries to conduct research or to speak, and has addressed audiences in her speeches and workshops ranging from Chinese military to Fortune 500 executives to high school teachers. She has been visiting professor at Rutgers, the State University of New Jersey, the Sorbonne, and the National Institute of Defense Studies of Japan, among others. She was a political commentator for over 20 years. She is the author of more than twenty books and forty articles on strategy. She is also a novelist, playwright, and visual artist.

INDEX

A

C

D

N

O

P

R

S

T

U

V

W